Health ~~Care~~ DARE!

8 Reasons to Try Natural Healing

By Monte Kline, Ph.D.

Published by:

Pacific Health Center
PO Box 1066
Sisters, OR 97759
www.pacifichealthcenter.com

ISBN - 13:978-1511948418

Copyright 2015 by Monte L. Kline

PUBLISHER'S NOTE: The information contained in this book is not intended for diagnosing illness or prescribing treatment. Rather the material herein is designed to be used in cooperation with your health practitioner to deal with personal health problems. Should you use this information on your own, you are prescribing for yourself, which is your constitutional right, but neither the author nor the publisher assumes responsibility.

Table of Contents

Introduction

I dare you. I dare you – not to do something stupid or dangerous -- but to do something that that may save your life – what I call a *health dare*:

I dare you to try natural healing

The "health dare" is no empty challenge, but rather one founded on eight solid reasons – eight reasons you should try natural healing.

In 1974 I took the "health dare" from a very unlikely source – an 80 year-old woman who changed my life. A couple months earlier a doctor told me at my ripe old age of 24 that I had cancer and required immediate surgery. Knowing next to nothing of alternative medicine, I consented, had surgery, and then consented again to five weeks of agonizing cobalt radiation therapy for possible spread of the disease that the diagnostic tests indicated had not spread.

It was then, as my days consisted of two divisions – throwing up and feeling like throwing up – that I received the "health dare" from my friend, Ada, who believed and was committed to nutritional cancer therapy. She filled my mailbox with big manila envelopes full of articles and tapes to support that conviction. Eventually, as I got sicker and sicker, she just wore me down.

I took the "health dare" by seeing a nutritionally-oriented M.D. she knew and that day began my "education" in natural healing, learning that I still had cancer (because my doctor had only been treating the symptoms, not the underlying cause of the disease) and that there was an effective natural healing approach. A year later I no longer had cancer and felt better than I had any time in my life. That "health dare" saved my life.

OVERCOMING BIASES

We all have our biases and preconceived notions of what's right and what's wrong, what truth is and what deception is. Those biases result from a lifetime of "inputs" that formed our convictions. Those inputs may have been true and legitimate or perhaps the opposite.

Part of the "health dare" is simply to temporarily lay aside the preconceived ideas you have about health care and be open to some new information – some new "inputs" upon which to base your beliefs. Here's the key question:

Will you consider eight reasons why you should try natural healing?

Will you just take a look at some facts and determine if this is for you – honestly decide if the possibility of natural healing is a "fit" for your situation? Will you consider the possibility that, whatever your particular health issues might be, a natural healing approach just might actually work for you?

THE KEY QUESTIONS

This is pretty simple and definitely not "rocket science." You need answers to a few key questions:

- Does natural healing work?
- Is it safe?
- Is it affordable?
- Can natural healing prevent future health problems?
- Will it be more comprehensive in dealing with my overall health?
- Can natural healing work with my conventional medical treatment?

This book will strive to answer those questions.

SPECIFIC HEALTH PROBLEMS

The purpose of this book is *not* to address *specific* health problems. I won't lay out a natural approach for your fatigue, depression, fibromyalgia, allergies, PMS, sinus issues or other problems. Many other books deal with those issues, as do I in my daily clinical practice, which is explained at the end of this book.

Rather, the approach of this book is simply to introduce you to a different philosophy of healing, particularly if you're a person who has never done a natural healing approach. My goal is to enable you to better decide if natural healing is an option for you. Will you take my "health dare" and carefully consider natural healing? That decision forever changed my life and health, and it can change yours as well.

I would hasten to add that although many health problems can be helped or resolved through natural healing approaches, not every problem can. But even if you're problem is not "fixable" through natural healing, generally natural healing methods help to some degree and can either complement your conventional treatment or even minimize negative side-effects of that treatment.

Let's see if I can make the case for natural healing. I dare you to try it.

Chapter 1

Natural Healing Works

Mr. Kline, you're in the Recovery Room. You have an oxygen tube in your nose. Just breathe normally.

I awoke to those words from a hospital nurse in September 1974 after having a cancerous tumor removed at the ripe old age of 24. It all happened so quickly – the lump, the pain, seeing a doctor and having him say, "You have cancer and we need to operate immediately." It was surreal. Up to that point I thought I was pretty healthy. I wasn't a big junk food eater. I even took some vitamins. Besides that, I felt good and had lots of energy. My perspective changed, however, with the announcement of cancer. For better and for worse my life would never be the same.

Natural healing alternatives? What's that? All I knew at that point was conventional, drug-oriented medicine, which I willingly submitted to. Within weeks I would begin to experience natural approaches to health care, but not before enduring some serious agony. You see, my situation didn't end with the surgical removal of that tumor. The next phase was five weeks of cobalt radiation therapy – therapy to supposedly stop further spread of the disease that all the diagnostic tests said had not spread. It's what I now call the "just in case" treatment.

I would go to the medical center for my out-patient appointments at 3:30 in the afternoon, get zapped for 40 seconds, get dressed and go home. Seems like no big deal. But, like clockwork day after agonizing day, at exactly 5:50 I would start throwing up and that would continue until 10:00 PM. There were just two divisions to my day – throwing up or feeling like throwing up. A depressing time? Absolutely. I didn't live in October 1974, I existed. And then God intervened with my first ***health dare***.

It's funny the way we so seldom recognize God's "arrival" to meet our needs. He so typically comes in unexpected forms. For me it was an 80 year-old woman, a supporter of our Christian ministry, who was convinced of natural alternatives for health problems. In retrospect, Ada didn't know a lot about health, but boy did she ever tell me everything she *did* know. A couple times a week I would receive big manila envelopes of literature and tapes on "nutritional cancer therapies." I did what any other thoroughly brainwashed health consumer would do and threw them away! Quackery! How could she be so deceived by all this nonsense!

Funny thing happened, though. As I got sicker and sicker on my "therapy," I became more open to health alternatives. And Ada was, if nothing else, persistent. She ultimately persuaded me to see a Christian medical doctor who was dealing with cancer patients from an alternative medicine perspective – I was, in effect, *dared* to try natural medicine. The day I saw him I began my education in the area of health. Like Mark Twain reportedly said:

> *I got my education all through my life . . . except for the years I was in school.*

I'll never forget that conversation:

> *Mr. Kline, the first thing I want to tell you is that you still have cancer. They've just been treating the symptom, but we need to deal with the underlying cause.*

He then laid out a program of dietary change, nutritional supplementation, immunotherapy, exercise, and intercessory prayer – a program that I strictly followed. My initial rather extensive nutritional supplement program was funded by a Christian family that skipped Christmas gifts to provide me with what I needed.

A year later there was no more cancer. I felt better than I had felt any time in my life in terms of energy and vitality. My main "problem" was a communication burden – I wanted others to know the principles of health I had learned. I started by teaching a lunch hour class at the Christian ministry where I worked. That led to writing my first book, leaving that Christian ministry, and presenting seminars in churches on biblical principles of health. Ultimately I completed a Ph.D. in Nutrition and went into clinical practice and continued to write books.

I share all this to let you know that I've been there. If you're struggling with a health problem and wondering about "health alternatives," I've been full circle on that subject. I've known the ignorance of natural health care, the doubts concerning effectiveness or safety, cost concerns and the like. The questions you have are the questions I intend to answer. Does natural healing work? It profoundly has for me. But let me tell the stories of others who dared to choose alternatives to conventional medicine.

KATHY – ANXIETY ATTACKS

One of my first clients after entering professional practice was a young mother suffering from anxiety attacks, medicated with heavy amounts of a highly addictive psychiatric drug. In desperation to help her, the Elders of her church sent her to me and paid for her initial testing. Here's how Kathy tells her story:

> *In December '84 I went to a local doctor and after an exam he said, "You might have an incurable disease and you don't want to have it." He didn't go into what the disease was or the treatments, but gave me a prescription and said come back in a month. Within four days I was in the hospital from an anxiety attack. My family doctor of 14 years refused to see me because I had gone to a specialist. A psychiatrist at the hospital said I needed tranquilizers, but physically I was fine – it was all mental. I was taking eight of them a day and climbing the walls. If I got dressed I was doing well. I knew if I had a physical the tests would be the same as in the hospital. If I was supposed to be physically okay, why was I feeling so terribly?*

Like many people, Kathy's anxiety problem was fundamentally iatrogenic – i. e. doctor-caused. How brutal and idiotic for a doctor to tell a patient they have an incurable disease and not say what the disease was. That would give anyone anxiety attacks! She then relates her experience hearing about my practice and coming into my clinic:

> *In January '85 I started their program. The tests they ran showed why I was feeling so badly. I was a mess. I followed their suggested diet and supplement program and within three months I was totally off the tranquilizers and had lost 35 pounds. I was able to care for my family again which meant so much for me. I can't tell you how good it felt to clean my house after months of not being able to. It is now July and I have lost altogether 51 pounds and am even working part-time . . . I'm so thankful to God for leading me here.*

Kathy told the story of her healing a lot – she became my Receptionist.

JOHN – ARTHRITIS

Would an 86 year-old blind widower crippled with arthritis take the "health dare" to try natural medicine? No, he didn't regain his sight as a result of natural healing. However, his main concern was arthritis in his hip that had required him to walk with a cane for the previous 20 years. After three days on an individualized diet and nutritional supplement program, he threw his cane away. After eight months he reported that his hip was fine. John tells part of his story this way:

> *When my hip was bothering me so badly I went to doctor after doctor and they never did help me! Some of them gave me pain shots and some wrote prescriptions out for me and charged me a lot more than you charge, and their methods didn't help at all, but yours did (and still do) . . . at 86 years of age I'm feeling better than I've felt in years and it's largely due to you and your work. Thanks!*

There was more to John's story, though. A few months after this, I heard that he had remarried!

MURIEL – HEADACHES & MORE

A lot of people who choose the alternative of natural healing have multiple health issues stealing a normal life from them, motivating them to take the natural health dare. Muriel was such a client:

> *My activities were down to 'zero' from a very active life . . . '300' blood pressure, damaged liver, organs and brain full of toxins, overweight, severe headaches, allergies to medications, severe all over rash, itching frenzies, and 40 years of chronic diarrhea. Then after two weeks of treatment my headaches were gone . . . also after two months my blood pressure was down to where I could drop most of that medication . . . I have lost 36 pounds and am very hopeful of fully recovering to a productive life again after just five months of treatment."*

Understand that she wasn't "treated" for any particular symptom or complaint. Instead, the underlying causes of her health issues were addressed so that roadblocks to healing would be removed. She took the "health dare" and changed her life.

DARLENE – TO BED AT 6 PM

Imagine your life if you had to rest four hours during the day and then go to bed at 6 PM because your fatigue was so severe. That was Darlene's situation – suffering for a year and half from bloating, cramps, diarrhea and debilitating fatigue. After seeking conventional medical help, she tried the health dare of natural medicine:

> *I was given a wide spectrum of tests by medical doctors that revealed nothing but good health. However, I was so weak and tired all the time and even depressed so the doctors gave me an antidepressant, which helped my emotions but made me physically worse . . . Then I came to see you, and after following your suggestions . . . in one week's time my bloating was gone, I had lost five pounds and my energy level had increased*

significantly. It has been two months now since that initial visit and I hardly ever need a nap, I have lost a total of ten pounds without ever feeling hungry, and I eased myself off the antidepressant and have been feeling great emotionally.

Unfortunately, it's all too common to be told by a conventional doctor, in spite of obvious and compelling symptoms, that there's nothing wrong with you . . . and then be sent to a psychiatrist! If you're sick, you really are sick, regardless of what any particular medical tests say. **If the "tests" don't explain your sickness, the problem is with the tests not you.**

KATHY – I GOT MY HUSBAND BACK

Sometimes the worst health problems we deal with are not our own, but rather those of a loved one we don't know how to help. Kathy saw her husband gradually withdrawing from life until he took the health dare:

I couldn't resist writing you to thank you for giving me back my husband. He was so severely plagued by depression that he had become suicidal and was retreating more and more into himself all the time. He recognized what was happening to himself and looked diligently to God's word and prayer to help find a way out. For years though he spent hours and hours in study and prayer and could not break free. Then we heard about your clinic through some friends and I convinced him to give it a try. Through the testing we found he had a need for lithium and that wheat was a major problem for him. That has been a little over a year ago and the change has been remarkable! . . . I remember after just a few weeks on the program he was given we heard him laugh for the first time in over three years. It brings tears to my eyes to think how wonderful it is to be able to talk to him and have him respond, to be able to look into his eyes and see life, not emptiness.

TAMI – 15 YEARS OF HEADACHES

Ever had a health problem so severe that you had to quit your job? Tami did:

> *I was desperate after suffering from daily headaches for 15 years. Along with the headaches, I was always tired and irritable and couldn't find the simple joy in life. I had exhausted all medical avenues after going through three months of tests with my doctor, who told me it was stress. So I quit my job and after two years was still having headaches every day. That's when I came to your clinic . . . After the initial testing I had mixed emotions. I was shocked to find out there were so many things going on in my body, but felt relieved to have answers. Finally, I felt validated. There was actually a reason for my headaches, fatigue and irritability. I went home determined to stay away from the 26 foods I was sensitive to, had vitamin and mineral supplements to deal with my deficiencies, and had tools to deal with the Candida and Chronic Fatigue Syndrome. By the next morning I was literally a new woman! The headaches were gone; I had joy in my heart and I was waking every morning at 5:15 fully refreshed and ready for another day. I don't know how to describe the vision improvements, the fog clearing out of my head, and the irritability disappearing. I have more patience for my kids and their fights . . . which I used to get right in the middle of. After less than a week my husband wanted an appointment just because of the difference he had seen in me . . . As an added bonus I've lost 20 pounds in six weeks . . . I praise God for teaching me to depend on Him for healing and for leading me to your clinic after the medical profession was unable to help me.*

All these people took the "health dare" and tried natural healing. They got answers, usually after previously getting nowhere with conventional, drug-oriented medicine. Of course, these are just a few examples from my practice. Other natural health care providers could share their own similar stories I'm sure. People don't go to alternative practitioners because they're stupid or brainwashed or delusional. They go simply because natural healing works.

NATURAL HEALING RESEARCH

It's not enough to *just* cite success stories of people helped by natural healing. Conventional medicine dismisses all that as "anecdotal," implying that the experience of real people is somehow inferior to results on lab rats. In other words, if it happened to a real human being, we really don't care, because we're smart and people are stupid or deceived!

The fact of the matter is that **lots** of scientific research has indeed validated natural healing approaches for many common health problems. Scientific studies are not the ultimate test, though, in that they too may be flawed. The combination of scientific research *and* repeated human experience makes the most compelling case for natural healing alternatives and can motivate you to take the health dare. Let's take a look at just a few common health problems and their scientifically validated natural approaches.

HIGH CHOLESTEROL

Conventional doctors routinely tell patients their cholesterol is too high and requires taking a cholesterol-lowering statin drug. As usual, they shoot the messenger that brings the bad news instead of reading the message. Why is the cholesterol high? Who knows – just take this $100 a month drug! Suspiciously, the norms for cholesterol keep changing downward opening a wider and wider market for what are already the most prescribed drugs today – the statins. Though *low* cholesterol can produce hormonal imbalances and even suicidal depression, people by the millions are told by ignorant doctors, "Your cholesterol can't be too low." Just take this drug.

Like all prescription drugs the statins have side-effects. After 31 people died from toxic reactions, the new cholesterol drug, Baychol, was withdrawn from the market in 2001.[1] Ironically, statins suppress the production of Coenzyme Q10 – one of the most important nutrients for cardiovascular health. Does it make sense to destroy one of the most important nutrients for heart health with a drug to supposedly help heart health?

Numerous natural remedies help high cholesterol with no side-effects – supplements such as fish oil, garlic and policosanol. Studies show that policosanol works as well as drugs for cholesterol lowering, yet sells for a fraction of the cost. Derived from sugar cane and without side-effects, it produces amazing results. In one six month double blind study, taking 20 mg of policosanol per day lowered LDL (the so-called "bad cholesterol") 27.4% and cholesterol itself by 15.6%. HDL (the so-called "good cholesterol") favorably increased by 17.6%.[2]

HIGH BLOOD PRESSURE

Hypertension is one of the most commonly medicated diseases, partly because of false positives on blood pressure at doctors' offices. So-called "white coat syndrome" raises many people's blood pressure – but only with the stress of being in a doctor's office! My mother was a very nervous, easily agitated person. She was put on an anti-hypertensive drug since her blood pressure was always high when the doctor checked it. But since that was a false positive, the drug made her blood pressure too low, resulting in fainting in church once until she stopped the drug she should have never been taking!

High blood pressure drugs manifest numerous side-effects. Generally they act as a diuretic, flushing out sodium. But they also flush out potassium which ironically is essential for the heart as well as other systems. Common drug side-effects include dizziness, drowsiness, blurred vision, headaches, gas, dry mouth, fatigue, stomach upset, difficulty breathing, and skin rash.

One of the natural healing approaches for hypertension is the antioxidant, coenzyme Q10. A study of 109 patients used 225 mg/day of CoQ10 and noted substantial improvement in blood pressure:

> *A definite and gradual improvement in function status was observed with the concomitant need to gradually decrease antihypertensive drug therapy within the first one to six months. Thereafter, clinical status and cardiovascular drug requirements stabilized with a significantly improved systolic and diastolic blood pressure.*

Most of the study participants (51%) were able to completely discontinue between one and three separate anti-hypertensive drugs on average after 4.4 months of taking CoQ10.[3]

Other research at the University of Chicago shows vitamin D to significantly affect high blood pressure.[4] Other researchers observe that hypertension is worse in winter than in the summer due to lack of ultraviolet light, which of course produces vitamin D as it reacts with the skin. Blood pressure progressively increases the farther one gets from the equator. The study also observes that Africans living in Europe have higher blood pressure than Africans living in Africa at the equator.[5] Study after study is now showing most people are deficient in vitamin D, in part due to the inadequate levels suggested from dietary and supplement sources. More significant supplementation of vitamin D (typically 4000 - 5000 units per day instead of 400 units) can greatly help high blood pressure and other problems.

PARKINSON'S DISEASE

Parkinson's disease is familiar to most people as central nervous system condition affecting motor skills and speech. Though often characterized by muscle tremors, it can also produce muscle rigidity or lack of movement altogether. Conventional medicine most often treats the symptoms with L-Dopa or related drugs. As always, side-effects and expense are an issue.

A 2003 Brazilian study found that of 31 consecutive Parkinson's patients, *all* were deficient in vitamin B-2. By contrast they found only three out of ten dementia patients deficient in this particular vitamin. Nineteen of the Parkinson's patients were put on 30 mg of B-2 per day along with eliminating red meat. After three months *all* showed improvement in motor skills capacity.[5]

ULCERS

Since the labeling in recent years of the *H. pylori* bacteria as the "cause" of ulcers, the condition has been treated primarily with antibiotic drugs. Antibiotics unfortunately compromise the immune system by destroying beneficial bacterial organisms in the gut as well. Would you believe that rhubarb is an alternative? A Chinese study of 64 ulcer patients involved treatment with 25 mg/kg of rhubarb per day. The rhubarb improved the stomach pH in the ulcer patients compared to the control group and reduced gastric bleeding by a whopping 73.4%![6] And of course the rhubarb costs little and has no side-effects.

DEPRESSION

Depression incidence has greatly increased with the decline of omega-3 fatty acids as found in fish, flaxseed, walnuts and other sources and the increase in omega-6 fatty acids as found in corn, safflower, sunflower, cottonseed, and sesame oils. While the *Journal of the American College of Nutrition* recommends a 1:1 ratio of omega-6 to omega-3, the average consumption in America is a 20:1 ratio, resulting in numerous health problems.[7,8,9] Dr. Joseph Hibbeln of the National Institutes of Health found that the higher a nation's consumption of fish, the lower the rate of depression.[10] He also discovered that higher fish consumption resulted both in less postpartum depression[11] and Seasonal Affective Disorder (SAD).[12]

BI-POLAR DISORDER

Bi-Polar refers to a depressive disorder characterized by either mania alone or mania alternating with depression, the latter being called "manic-depressive." Most often conventional medicine treats Bi-Polar Disorder with prescription lithium carbonate. The drug has significant side-effects, in part due to proximity of the therapeutic and toxic levels of lithium. But are there natural alternatives?

A four month, double-blind, placebo-controlled study compared fish oil (omega 3 fatty acids) as compared to olive oil as a control with bi-polar patients. The fish oil group had significantly longer remission than the placebo group and also performed better on every other outcome measured.[13] Which would you rather use – a lithium drug or fish oil?

MULTIPLE SCLEROSIS (MS)

MS is another progressive, neuromuscular disease, characterized by the loss of the myelin sheath around the nerves. This results in a wide range of symptoms including muscle movement issues, balance, speech, fatigue, depression, cognitive ability, and others. Conventional medicine uses various drugs in an attempt to control symptoms, but not without significant side-effects.

A study at the Oregon Health & Sciences University found Ginkgo Biloba herb effective in helping MS. Ginkgo is known particularly for increasing circulation, especially cerebral circulation. Of 39 people in the study, 20 received Ginkgo, while 19 received a placebo. The Ginkgo group performed 13% faster on a timed color and word test (Stroop Test) that measure attention, planning, decision making, controlling goal-directed behavior and executing deliberate actions. Improvements were also noted in fatigue and muscle pain. A survey of 1913 MS patients in Oregon found that 20% used Ginkgo and 39% of those found it beneficial for their symptoms.[14] Those who suffer from a disease aren't stupid – they do what works.

ASTHMA

Asthma can be a terrifying problem. To go without food or water is one thing, but to be unable to breathe is quite another. Conventional doctors prescribe oral drugs for chronic symptoms and inhalers for acute symptoms. Thankfully there are effective medications for the emergency asthma attacks, but what about actually solving the underlying causes?

One of many successful natural healing approaches employs Butterbur Root herb. In a study of 80 patients with mild to moderate asthma, two-thirds had improved airflow after two months of taking 50 – 150 mg per day of the herb. Again we have a healing method that's natural, side-effect free and cheap.[15]

MIGRAINES

Typical migraine sufferers choose between regular episodes of debilitating headaches or being heavily medicated with toxic drugs. The herb, Butterbur, again helps this health problem. In this study 245 migraine sufferers received either Butterbur or a placebo twice a day. A 48% reduction in symptoms was noted with the Butterbur group, whereas there was just a 26% reduction with the placebo group who thought they were being medicated.[16]

BREAST CANCER

I could cite many examples of documentation of natural healing for cancer, but will only cite one very simple finding. A study confirmed that oleic acid, the primary monounsaturated fatty acid found in olive oil, promotes the death of breast cancer cells through an immune stimulation pathway.[17]

ALZHEIMER'S DISEASE

All diseases are terrible, but Alzheimer's is uniquely cruel in slowly bringing mental death to those still physically alive. I know, since my father died of the disease. Perhaps more than with any other disease, the family caregivers experiences the results of the disease more than the no longer cognizant victim. The conventional medical approach is rather bleak, mostly offering highly liver toxic drugs that do not significantly affect symptoms. But what about natural healing?

Researchers at UCLA found that the brain needs fish oil to make a plaque fighting protein. Greg M. Cole, Ph.D., Associate Director of the UCLA Alzheimer's Disease Research Center states the people who get plenty of DHA (docosahexaenoic acid) from fish oil have a reduced risk of developing Alzheimer's.[18]

The herb, curcumin, also appears to fight the plaque development on the brain characteristic of Alzheimer's disease. Curcumin is the yellow pigment found in curry spice, common in Indian cuisine. The *Journal of Biological Chemistry* reported that curcumin was as effective as many other Alzheimer's drugs in preventing brain plaques. Furthermore, they found it to actually break up existing plaques.[19] Curcumin medicinal usage in India dates back thousands of years.

Another herbal remedy extensively used for Alzheimer's and other forms of dementia is Huperzine A, derived from Chinese club moss. Over 100,000 people in China have been treated with this herbal remedy. Research at the Shanghai Institute of Materia Medica found Huperzine A more effective than common Alzheimer's drugs in facilitating memory improvement.[20] In a study fifty Alzheimer's patients received 200 mcg of Huperzine A twice a day for eight weeks. Of the 50, 29 showed improvement in memory, cognitive and behavior abilities.[21]

The B vitamin, folic acid, may also offer help to those with dementia symptoms. South Korean researchers monitored 518 elderly persons who did not have dementia, tracking them over a period of 2.4 years. During the study, 45 had developed dementia, including 34 who were diagnosed with Alzheimer's disease. Specifically they found that decreased levels of folic acid were associated with increased onset of dementia.[22]

Yet another natural remedy for memory problems is phosphatidyl serine (PS). Numerous studies indicate significant cognitive improvement using this supplement. One study using the now preferred plant source PS showed positive effects on daily functioning, emotional state and self-reported general condition of Alzheimer's patients. After this relatively short, two-month study, nearly half the participants were sufficiently convinced of the value of the supplement that they decided to continue it at their own expense.[23] Since other studies on PS indicate six months usage is required to observe substantial benefits, improvement in just two months is very impressive.

These are but a few of the examples that could be cited of solid scientific research documenting the effectiveness of natural healing for common health problems. So many simple items – foods, herbs, vitamins, minerals – can so profoundly impact our health. It is no longer a matter of accepting perhaps subjective testimonial evidence about health alternatives. More and more the hard science is validating these simple and effective approaches.

BUT WHY DOES IT WORK?

I guess the next question is simply, "Why does natural healing work?" If you've only experienced conventional, drug-oriented health care your whole life, it may come as quite a surprise that **natural healing actually works!** Here's the simple reason: Natural healing works because it is *consistent* with God's design of the body, rather than *competitive* as drug approaches are. To put it another way, natural healing encourages the body, while drug healing fights with the body.

The effective approach of natural healing can be summarized with two questions:

> (1) What's *missing* in my body that *should* be there?

> (2) What's *present* in my body that *should not* be there?

"What's missing" concerns nutrient deficiencies. "What's present" includes toxins and allergic sensitivities. Regardless of the specific health problem, the "common denominators" of deficiencies, toxicity and sensitivity will usually be factors. A natural healing approach that eliminates toxins and allergens and adds needed nutrients is bound to work to at least some degree. Aligning with God's design produces results, as we'll discuss in more detail in the last chapter.

Abundant evidence demonstrates the *effectiveness* of natural healing, but what about *safety*? Before you commit to the "health dare," you need assurance of safety. We tackle this question next.

CHAPTER ONE FOOTNOTES

1. Hodgson J., Bayer lapse exposes pharm's vulnerability. *Nat Biotechnol* 2001 Oct;19(10)897-8.

2. Castana G, et al. Effects of policosanol 20 versus 40 mg/day in the treatment of patients with type II hypercholesterolemia: a 6-month double-blind study. *Int J Clin Pharmacol Res* 2001;21(1):43-57.

3. Langsjoen P, Langsjoen P, Willis R, Folkers K, Treatment of essential hypertension with coenzyme Q10, *Mol Aspects Med.* 1997;15 Supple:dS265-72.

4. Li YC, Qiao G, Uskokovic M, Xiang W, Zheng W, Kong J, Vitamin D: a negative endocrine regulator of the rein-angiotensin system and blood pressure. *J Steroid Biochem Mol Biol.* 2004 May;89-90(1-5):387-392.

5. Coimbra CG, Junqueira VBC, High doses of riboflavin and the elimination of dietary red meat promote the recovery of some motor function in Parkinson's disease patients. *Braz J Med Biol Res* 2003;36:1409-1417.

6. Zhongguo Zhong Xi Yi Jie He Za Zhi, 2000 July;20(7):515-8.

7. Simopoulos AP, Leaf A, Salem N, Workshop on the essentiality of and recommended dietary intakes for omega-6 and omega-3 fatty acids. *J Am Coll Nutr* 1999; 18:487-489.

8. Simopoulos AP, Evolutionary aspects of diet and essential fatty acids. *World Rev Nutr Diet* 2001; 88:18-27.

9. Simopoulos AP, Evolutionary aspects of n-3 fatty acids in the diet. *World Rev Nutr Diet* 1998; 83:1-11.

10. Hibbeln JR, Fish consumption and major depression. *Lancet* 1998; 351:1213.

11. Hibbeln JR, Seafood consumption, the DHA content of mothers milk and prevalence rates of postpartum depression: a cross-natioonal, ecological analysis. *J Affect Disord* 2002; 69:15-29.

12. Cott J, Hibbeln JR, Lack of seasonal mood change in Icelanders. *Am J Psychiatry* 2001;158:328.

13. Stoll AL, Severus WE, Freeman MP, Rueter S et al. Omega 3 fatty acids in bipolar disorder: a preliminary double-blind, placebo-controlled trial. *Arch Gen Psychiatry* 1999 May;56(5):407-12.

14. Oregon Health & Science University (2005, April 28). OHSU Study Finds Ginkgo Beneficial For MS Symptoms. *SCIENCEDAILY*. Retrieved November 20, 2008, from http://www.sciencedaily.com /releases/2005/04/050428093022.htm.

15. Danesch U. Petasites hybridus (Butterbur root) extract in the treatment of asthma an open trial. *Altern Med Rev* 2004;9(1):54-62.

16. Brown RP and Gerbarg PL, Herbs and nutrients in the treatment of depression, anxiety, insomnia, migraine, and obesity. *J Psychiatr Pract* 2001 Mar;7(2):75-91.

17. Menendez JA Vellon L, Colomer R Lup R Oleic acid, the main monounsaturated fatty acid of olive oil, suppresses Her-2/neu (erbB-2) expression and synergistically enhances the growth inhibitory effects os trastuzumab (Herceptin) in breast cancer cells with Her-2/neu oncogene amplication, *Ann Oncol* 2005 Mar;16(3):339-40.

18. DeNoon Daniel J, Fish oil prevents Alzheimer's plaques, Dec. 26, 2007, http://www.webmd.com/alzheimers/news/2007/1226/fish-oil-prevents-alzheimers-plaques.

19. *J Biol Chem*, Dec. 7, 2004, online edition.

20. *Neuroreport* 1996, Dec. 20; 8(1):97-101.

21. Chung Kuo Yao Li Hsueh Pao 1995, Sept; 116(5)391-395.

22. Kim J, Stewart R, Kim S, Shin I, Yang S, Shin H, Yoon, J, Changes in folate, vitamin B12 and homocysteine associated with incident dementia. *J Neurol*, published online ahead of print, doi 10.1136/jnnp.2007.131482.

23. Gindin J, et. Al. 1990, Effect of soy lecithin phosphatidylserine (PS) treatment on daily function and self-reported general condition in patients with Alzheimer's disease, The Geriatric Institute of Education and Research, Kaplan Medical Centre, Rehovot, and Hadassah Medical School, Hebrew University of Jerusalem, Israel.

Chapter 2

Natural Healing is Safe

Well, I sure would never go to one of those "kwhyros!"

Growing up in Illinois just across the Mississippi from the largest chiropractic college in the country, everybody had an opinion about those "kwhyros," as they were often diminutively called. And, oh the talk about someone who "health dared" to go see one those "kwhyros" -- why they were really taking a big risk with their health! Though a lot of people saw chiropractors with great success, as a kid it seemed to me that most thought that health alternative was somewhere between weird and satanic. Understand that most of those folks couldn't even pronounce "chiropractic," but they *knew* it was something dangerous and to be feared. The same people had complete confidence is driving a few hours north to the Mayo Clinic in Rochester, while never giving the slightest thought to the safety of *conventional* medicine.

Though I grew up with that prejudice against chiropractic, neck and back pain eventually dissolved my fears enough to see my first chiropractor at age 23. With a few simple adjustments I was feeling much better and have kept chiropractic as a big part of my personal health care ever since. As far as I know, I am the only person in even my extended family that has ever been to a chiropractor, much less any other kind of alternative health practitioner. Unbelievable!

Do you feel "safe" with conventional medicine and maybe a little "fearful" of natural healing? You're not alone. People often approach a health alternative with one of two emotions – skepticism or fear. In the first chapter we dealt with the unjustified skepticism, while in this chapter we deal with the similarly inappropriate fear. Is natural healing really safe? Will a natural healing approach give me yet another health problem? Will I experience harm from doing a natural method and thus delaying implementation of conventional medicine for my problem?

These questions must be answered before you'll be willing to take the "health dare" into natural healing. No matter how convinced you may be of the *effectiveness* of natural healing, your greater concern (and rightly so) is *safety.*

To one degree or another we're all brainwashed on many subjects, not the least of which is health. Our beliefs reflect the inputs we have received and accepted. Positive inputs produce feelings of safety, while negative inputs breed suspicion and fear. If the media, schools, doctors, parents, friends and the like have all planted and watered suspicion and fear over natural healing, we will automatically think that way. The gigantic economic interests of the conventional medicine-drug industry naturally want to keep you buying their products and services. Therefore, they will do everything they can to keep you from the "competition" through misinformation. They don't want you to place any trust in natural healing alternatives that cost them business. I'm not being crass here – that's just reality.

The irony of this state of affairs is bizarre. The people most concerned about the safety of natural healing usually never even question the safety of conventional medicine. Yet, as we will see in this chapter, **conventional medicine is one of the greatest *proven* threats to your health!** People should be screaming about the safety issues with medical treatment, not with vitamins and other natural remedies. Nevertheless, we must maintain a balanced approach that recognizes the benefits and the cautions of both conventional and natural healing. Simply stated, we must abandon the propaganda and seek out the truth.

NATURAL HEALING MISINFORMATION

There's an old saying in the news business that "if it bleeds, it leads." The more violent, shocking or fantastic the story, the more attention it draws, and the more readers or viewers it attracts. Thus contrary studies always make page one, no matter how off the wall they are compared to established knowledge. Here's an example from the June 15, 2001 UK *Daily Mail*:

> *Vitamin C Cancer Fear – High Doses of Vitamin C Could Increase the Risk of Cancer.*

The operative word here is "could." The study referred to failed to show that high doses of vitamin C did cause cancer, but that's what the average person would take away from the article. Nor did the article highlight the large amount of existing data supporting the benefits of vitamin C for health issues including cancer.

The study in question is by Dr. Ian Blair, resident researcher at the University of Pennsylvania Pharmacology Unit. Though Dr. Blair seemingly contradicted that headline by saying, "Absolutely, for God's sake, don't say Vitamin C causes cancer,"[1] the reporting of his study certainly gave that impression. Blair theorizes that high amounts of vitamin C, as beneficially used for decades in non-toxic cancer therapies, might cause tissue degeneration, which in turn could lead to more cancer.

On closer examination the study loses merit. Vitamin C was combined in a test tube with substances formed in the oxidation of saturated fats (lipid hydroperoxides) which resulted in the production of compounds that can damage DNA. Sounds like a real problem until you get the experiment out of the test tube and into a living human body. This effect cannot happen in the body due to enzyme systems that remove the damaging substances. Furthermore, vitamin E in living systems protects cells from this oxidation encouraged by vitamin C – the very nutrient being called the villain. It's an interesting study for chemistry class, but highly misleading for evaluating issues of human health.

DOES VITAMIN E SHORTEN LIFESPAN?

Another study by Edgar Miller, MD of Johns Hopkins concluded that taking 400 IU of vitamin E increases the risk of dying by 10%! It further surmised that vitamin E doesn't really protect the heart.[2] This was not an original study, but rather the re-evaluation of 19 previous studies – which is where the problem begins. Annette Dickinson, Ph.D., President of the Council for Responsible Nutrition notes that 18 of the 19 studies showed no significant mortality increase from taking vitamin E. However, putting all 19 studies together significantly skews the data.[3]

But that's only part of the problem. All 19 studies evaluated involved people already sick with heart disease or cancer or Alzheimer's disease. That fact obviously introduces many more variables as compared to evaluating the effect of vitamin E on healthy individuals. Dr. Dickinson notes:

> The definitive study to test vitamin E in a healthy population has not been done.

Dr. Walter Willett, Chairman of the Department of Nutrition at Harvard School of Public Health echoes this thought regarding vitamin E studies:

> I don't think we have the final answer.

He notes that women receiving vitamin E in the Women's Health Study had a 24% *decrease* in cardiovascular disease mortality.[4] Many other studies similarly show great health benefits from vitamin E. However, without the full information, paranoia over the safety of natural healing methods inevitably results.

WHY THE PROPAGANDA?

The above studies are but two examples of hundreds that could be cited that reach rather misleading conclusions – all factors that *demotivate* you from taking the health dare of trying natural healing approaches. But why does such a regular pattern of trashing natural healing approaches exist? I always say that when all else fails, follow the money. A University of Manchester publication on research methodology notes:

> Science and research must be studied in the context of all the interested parties involved. The questions center on determining the relative weight of the various allies in the "fact-creating" process – e.g. funding bodies, businesses, departments of state, professions and other scientists. In analyzing scientific debates, one should always ask what social, institutional, political and philosophical interests lie behind often apparently "neutral" and "technical" knowledge claims.[5]

For example, it's interesting to note the funding of the University of Pennsylvania Cancer Center referred to earlier. This institution is funded by the National Institutes of Health, the National Cancer Institute, the American Cancer Society, the Leukemia Society, and many pharmaceutical companies. In other words, they are funded by the conventional cancer treatment establishment. Would that have an effect on the evaluation of an alternative modality for helping cancer, such as vitamin C? You decide.

STUDIES: CAN YOU TRUST THEM?

Most people trust scientific studies. Most scientists and doctors worship them. Yet are scientific studies the be-all, end-all of truth? Hardly. The barrage of conflicting findings from such research is familiar to anyone that's watched TV or read a newspaper. Coffee's bad for you; coffee's good for you. Saturated fats are bad for you; saturated fats are good for you. Eggs are bad for your cholesterol; eggs are fine. Milk is good for you; milk is the worst thing you can put in our body. And on and on it goes. What do you believe?

The real question is whether one can squeeze truth into the confines of a study. Unfortunately for research scientists, truth is often not that malleable. A false premise underlies most scientific studies, namely that you can isolate a question down to one variable and test only that. For example, in the earlier studies cited researchers wanted to know if vitamin C helped or hurt cancer. They proceeded to experiment in a test tube, the result of which was proving only what happens in a test tube. The human body is far more complex with multitudes of other variables such as the enzyme production that makes what happened in the test tube impossible to happen in a living body.

Suppose we wanted to do a study on whether people who take vitamins live longer. It's not a problem to divide people into two groups – those that take vitamins and those that don't – and track lifespan. But what about all the other variables in the lives of the study participants? Maybe the people that take vitamins also do a lot of other things not done by the non-vitamin group: eating better, exercising, not smoking, maybe more safety conscious, etc. Can you really screen out all those other variables to get a true result? That's somewhere between difficult and impossible.

Vitamin C pioneer, Linus Pauling, Ph.D., though the only man to win two unshared Nobel prizes, was often critical of false conclusions from scientific studies. He once described a hypothetical study to determine if calcium strengthened the bones. Cannon balls would be dropped from a 100 foot tower onto the skulls of two participants, one who had taken calcium supplements and one who had not. Since both had their skulls crushed by the cannon balls, the study concluded that calcium was of no benefit in strengthening the bones! A lot of scientific studies are structured almost like that.

Don't get me wrong, for I'm not saying we should quit doing scientific studies. I am saying we should not fall down and worship them as the ultimate truth about health (or anything else). A lot of things cannot be proven by a scientific study. **Life is larger than a laboratory!** Ultimate truth is revealed, not "studied," being revealed in God's word, in God's creation, in the human heart, and in plain old common sense. One should keep in mind the bigger view of the forest and not get too myopic looking at the trees. Truth will ultimately be confirmed in human experience rather than a test tube.

NATURAL HEALING SAFETY

Let me begin this core question of safety by asking this:

> Have you ever heard of someone dying from a natural healing method?

> Do you even know anyone who has heard of anyone thus losing their life?

Probably not. But let me then ask another question:

Have you ever heard of someone dying from conventional medical treatment?

I'll bet you have. How many people die in the operating room? How many die from prescription drug reactions? How many die from other medical mistakes? I'll tell you in a moment. But how many actually die from natural healing methods? The Centers for Disease Control (CDC) has published statistics on the top 113 causes of death in the U. S. Looking down the list I note that malignant neoplasms (cancer) in 2005 killed 559,312 people, while cardiovascular diseases killed 856,030.[5] But you know, I looked and looked down that list and couldn't find any natural healing modalities in the top 113 causes of death. Overdosing on vitamins (hypervitaminosis) was not listed. Chiropractic adjustments or massage therapy were not listed. Acupuncture was not listed. Reactions to homeopathic or herbal medicines was likewise not listed. One would think, with all the paranoia in the media over health alternatives, that surely these natural healing methods must be a significant cause of death. But they are not.

Let's focus on one of the most basic natural healing approaches – taking vitamins. How safe is it to take vitamins? After all, aren't doctors always telling us not to take high doses of vitamins? Aren't they always telling us, "You get all the vitamins you need in the food you eat?" Of course most doctors don't really believe that when it comes to taking vitamins themselves. For example, a survey of 4501 doctors in the Women Physicians Health Study revealed that half of them took a multi-vitamin.[6] I guess it's "Do as I say, not as I do." But back to the question, "How safe is vitamin therapy?"

A 24 year review by the American Association of Poison Control Centers notes the following:[7]

Vitamins are among the 16 most reported substances to their centers

In 16 of the 24 years there was not a single death from taking vitamins

The other years had either one or two deaths attributed to vitamin usage

In 24 years only 11 people in the U. S. were killed by vitamins

So how does that compare to annual deaths by other substances and causes:

Aspirin – 59 deaths

Acetaminophen – 147 deaths

Aerosol air fresheners – 2 deaths

Table salt – 1 death

Baking soda – 1 death

Perfume/cologne/aftershave – 2 deaths

Let me add one more: There are an average of 54 deaths per year from lightning.[8] Imagine that! You are 54 times more likely to be struck by lightning and killed than to die from taking vitamins!

Zero to two deaths per year from vitamins, in spite of the fact that:

Half of all Americans take vitamins daily

That represents 145 million individual doses daily

Therefore 53 billion doses of vitamins annually

That's a lot of vitamins to only produce zero to two deaths per year.

ACUPUNCTURE SAFETY

Acupuncture is an increasingly common natural healing method that has been extensively studied for safety. The *British Medical Journal* reported on a study of 34,000 acupuncture treatments by 548 British acupuncturists (31% of the acupuncturists in the entire country). Not only were there no deaths in 34,000 treatments, but there were only minor reactions reported. It concluded:

There were no reports of serious adverse events, defined as events requiring hospital admission, leading to permanent disability, or resulting in death.[9]

Natural healing is not just safe, but it is amazingly safe compared to almost anything you do in life. Now why don't you ever hear about this in the media? You certainly hear as a lead story every bit of obscure, ill-conceived research lambasting some vitamin or herb. Is there an agenda in play here? Is perhaps anti-natural healing publicity a diversion from the greater issue of the dangers of conventional medicine?

DEADLY DOCTORS

The real question is not, "Is natural healing safe?" but rather, "Is conventional medicine safe?" Numerous studies of iatrogenic (doctor-caused) disease reveal an alarming safety problem. While the media focuses on anti-vitamin research, it mostly ignores blatant findings of widespread doctor-caused disease.

So, who says so? How about the *Journal of the American Medical Association* for one. According to Barbara Starfield, MD of the Johns Hopkins School of Hygiene and Public Health, **conventional medical treatment is the third leading cause of death in America**, after cardiovascular disease and cancer. Dr. Starfield's research, published in the July 26, 2000 issue of JAMA notes the following annual "doctor-caused" deaths[10]:

12,000 – Unnecessary Surgery

7,000 – Prescription medication errors

20,000 – Other hospital errors

80,000 – Hospital acquired infections

106,000 –No-Error, Negative Effects of Drugs

225,000 – TOTAL IATROGENIC DEATHS

Bet you never heard that on the evening news!

DOCTORS VS. GUNS

Just for fun, let's compare deaths by doctors to deaths by firearms. Consider these numbers:

700,000 Medical doctors in the U. S.

225,000 Doctor-caused deaths/year

That equals 1 death for every 3 doctors

80,000,000 gun owners in the U. S.

1,000 accidental deaths/year

That equals 1 death for every 80,000 gun owners

Therefore doctors are 26,000 times more dangerous than guns!

DELAYED TREATMENT QUESTION

One of the most frequent complaints lodged against natural healing is that it delays conventional medical treatment. Critics of natural healing gravely warn that if you waste time with a natural healing method instead of immediately running to conventional medicine, it may cost you your life. Of course, there's no evidence of this, nor could there be – how could we know for sure what would happen "if" we made a different treatment choice? This is strictly supposition.

However, the doctor-caused disease research would actually suggest just the opposite conclusion: If conventional medical treatment is killing 225,000 people per year, one might logically assume the healthiest course of action would be to avoid such treatment in order to extend life. For conventional doctors to try to keep people in conventional medicine and out of natural healing for safety reasons is like someone encouraging you to take up bull riding because it's safer than bird watching! Based on the evidence, trying *conventional* medicine should be a whole lot more of a "health dare" than trying natural healing.

DOCTORS REFUSE THEIR OWN MEDICINE

Many years ago my wife and I took the jet "Mail Boat" trip up the Rogue River in Southern Oregon. As one of the men from the boat company brought the mail bag for delivery to the Agness Post Office 30 miles upriver, a lady on the boat said, "Aren't you coming with us?" He pointed to our pilot saying, "Ride with that guy? Are you kidding?" Of course that was a joke probably doled out to every boat load of tourists that left the dock. But it's not much different when your doctor wouldn't personally use the treatments he recommends for you. You have to ask if you would:

Eat food at a restaurant that its cook refuses to eat

Buy a Ford from a car dealer that only drives Chevys himself

Buy any product from someone who won't use it themselves

Yet people do just that with doctors – at least when it comes to cancer.

McGill Cancer Center surveyed experts on lung cancer to ascertain which of six current conventional therapies they would use if they had cancer. Out of 79 respondents 64 of them said they would refuse cis-platinum, a common chemotherapy drug – 81% of them wouldn't do that chemotherapy that they repeatedly recommended to their patients. It gets worse though, in that 58 of the 79 oncologists (73%) said they wouldn't use any of the six therapies due to ineffectiveness or toxicity.[11] Professor Gorge Mathe stated:

> *If I were to contract cancer, I would never turn to a certain standard for the therapy of this disease. Cancer patients who stay away from these centers have some chance to make it.*[12]

I don't have much confidence in a healing approach doctors wouldn't use themselves. Herein we define a major difference between conventional and natural healing: People seldom become medical doctors because of positive experiences with their own health using conventional medicine. However, most people in natural healing (including myself) pursued that field precisely because of the personal results we experienced. Thus you're less likely to have a natural healing practitioner say, "Do as I say, not as I do" simply because he *is* doing what he's telling you to do.

Maybe the first question to ask your doctor regarding a proposed treatment is:

Would you use this approach yourself?

If not, it may be time to look for a health alternative.

DRUG INTERFERENCE?

Does natural healing interfere with the action of drugs? In some cases the answer is "yes," but I would have to ask, "How is that necessarily a bad thing?" Dr. Starfield's study cited earlier, notes that over 100,000 Americans die every year from non-error prescription drug reactions. So could we not assume that lives would be saved by "interfering" with the action of those drugs? That argument could be made.

Obviously when a drug is being taken for a specific medical reason, there could be a problem if some natural remedy is counteracting that medication. For example, if you're having an organ transplant, it's essential to avoid any immune stimulating remedies, perverse as that might seem. Likewise, if you're about to have surgery, you don't really want vitamin E or other natural remedies thinning your blood. These are, of course, very unusual and exceptional situations.

On the other hand one might argue that if you were using the natural healing modality first, perhaps you wouldn't need that conflicting drug or extreme medical procedures. So why is the natural remedy always assumed to be the interloper on the healing process? Why is it the "bad guy" that needs to be eliminated? For example, I've often had clients taking Warfarin (Coumadin$_{TM}$) from their M.D. that were told not to take vitamin E. The logic is simple: Warfarin thins the blood and so does vitamin E, so they don't want your blood to get too thin. Okay, I get it – you shouldn't be taking two blood thinning remedies. But why should the $10 - $20/month vitamin E be cast aside in favor of the $70/month Warfarin? Could it be because the vitamin E manufacturer isn't spending $5,000 a year wining and dining your medical doctor with free samples, trips to Hawaii, and the like?

But I truly believe the bias is about more than just slick marketing by drug company salesmen. Conventional medicine is the establishment healing art, if you will the "alpha male" that sees all other healing approaches as secondary. Like all alpha males, it asserts the right to eat first at the trough. In its view it is supreme and will destroy those who do not defer to its primacy, as most health practitioners who seriously challenge conventional medicine soon discover.

Nowhere is my admonition to "follow the money" more appropriate than here. In this whole process I've been describing there is one conspicuous omission – the patient. If the patient's benefit were indeed the main concern, they would be told to take vitamin E instead of Warfarin at a fraction of the cost. If the patient's benefit were the primary concern there would be a lot less drugs prescribed by medical doctors and a lot more herbs, vitamins, minerals, enzymes and amino acids. Conventional medicine has become more about marketing a product profitably than about healing. Part of that marketing plan is suppressing competition, whether by media misinformation, legislative or legal action.

NATURAL HEALING CAUTIONS

In discussing the problems and perversions of conventional medicine I do not want to give the impression that you should have no concerns whatever with natural healing. First of all, judgment is required to make good health decisions, whether you're using conventional medicine, natural healing or both in combination. You need to know the facts on the issues concerning your health. Get as much information as possible from as many sources and perspectives as possible. The internet functions as an amazing resource in this regard. A well informed "health consumer" will not be a victim of propaganda. After you're well informed, just use common sense.

Secondly, absolutely do not reject all conventional medicine. We all need conventional medicine, though not necessarily for every health problem. We also all need natural healing, though not necessarily for every health problem. Both approaches have limitations and biases. Recognize those limitations. Be alert to those biases. Ideally your health strategy should feature conventional and natural healing in a complementary relationship. We'll cover that in detail in a later chapter.

Thirdly, realize that there are interactions between some natural remedies and some prescription drugs. I emphasize "some" simply because there are no conflicts with most natural remedies. Most of the conflicts occur with herbal remedies. If it is absolutely not possible for you to transition off a prescription medication in favor of a natural remedy, you need to keep the following possible herb-drug interactions taken from the *Merck Manual* in mind[13]:

Anticoagulants (Warfarin, etc.)

> Contraindicated Herbs: Chamomile, Feverfew, Garlic, Ginger, Ginkgo, Ginseng
>
> Interaction: May increase risk of bleeding
>
> Contraindicated Herbs: Goldenseal, St. John's Wort
>
> Interaction: May increase risk of blood clots

Barbiturates

> Contraindicated Herbs: Chamomile, St. John's Wort, Valerian
>
> Interaction: May increase sedative effect

Immunosuppressants

> Contraindicated Herbs: Echinacea
>
> Interaction: Immune stimulation, may counteract immune suppression

Hypoglycemic drugs (insulin, glipizide, etc.)

> Contraindicated Herbs: Garlic, Ginseng, Milk Thistle
>
> Interaction: May increase blood sugar lowering effect

MAO inhibitor Antidepressants

Contraindicated Herbs: Ginkgo, Ginseng

Interaction: May increase effect of drug antidepressant or produce headaches, tremors, manic episodes

Contraindicated Herb: St. John's Wort

Interaction: May increase effect of drug or cause very high blood pressure

Selective serotonin Reuptake Inhibitors – SSRI's (Fluoxetine, paroxetine, sertraline, etc.)

Contraindicated Herb: St. John's Wort

Interaction: May increase effect of these reuptake inhibitors

Antihypertensives & Antiarrhythmics

Contraindicated Herb: Licorice

Interaction: May increase blood pressure and risk of arrhythmia

Non-Steroidal Anti-Inflammatories (NSAIDs)

Contraindicated Herb: Feverfew

Interaction: Drugs reduce effectiveness of Feverfew in managing migraines

Whether the above *possible* interactions are a problem or not depends upon your perspective: Are the drugs the "bad guy" or are the herbal remedies the "bad guy?" If you have no alternative and must take those drugs, you need to beware of the conflicts the natural remedies might present. However, if you are able to use a natural approach such that you don't need to take the conflicting drugs, the interactions are of no concern. In fact, you'll probably be delighted to know that an inexpensive herb has similar actions to a more expensive and side-effect laced drug.

Let's go back to our original question, "Is natural healing safe?" I would answer that question with a "Yes, but . . ." Compared to conventional medicine, natural healing by any measure is extremely safe. But natural healing does require knowledge and common sense to use it properly. Natural healing can most definitely be abused. My advice is to get good information both from your own research and from qualified and experienced natural health care providers as well as conventional medical practitioners. Then you can make the best health decisions utilizing both conventional and natural healing.

Does the safety of natural healing motivate you to take the "health dare?" I hope so, but let's look at another motivating factor – cost.

CHAPTER TWO FOOTNOTES

1. Ransom, Steven, "More On the Concern Over Vitamin C: Oh Yes? And Who's 'They'?, **www.whatareweswallowing.com** and from July 2001 Campaign for Truth in Medicine at **www.campaignfortruth.com**.

2. Miller, Edgar R III, et. al., "Meta-Analysis: High-Dosage Vitamin E Supplementation May Increase All-Cause Mortality," *Annals of Internal Medicine* 142(1) January 4, 2005.

3. "CRN Urges Caution in Weighing Results of New Vitamin E Study," **http://nutrition.about.com/od/researchstudies/a/vitaminecrn.htm** .

4. "What Vitamins Do Doctors Take and Why?" **http://www.happyhealthylonglife.com/happy_healthy_long_life/2008**

5. University of Manchester Institute of Science & Technology (UMIST) research methodology course handout, 1994.

6. "Number of Deaths from 113 Selected Causes by Age: United States, 2005, Centers for Disease Control.

7. American Association of Poison Control Centers, **http://www.aapcc.org/Annual%20Reports/03report/Annual%20Report%202003.pdf**

8. **http://www.lightningsafety.com/nlsi)lls/fatalities_us.html**

9. MacPherson H, Thomas K, Walters S, Fitter M, The York acupuncture safety study: prospective survey of 34,000 treatments by traditional acupuncturists, *British Medical Journal* 2001;323;486-487.

10. Starfield B, JAMA July 26, 2000;284(4)483-5.

11. Day, Philip, **Cancer: Why We're Still Dying to Know the Truth**, Credence Publications, 2000.

12. Mathe, Gorge, Scientific Medicine Stymied, Medicines Nouvelles, Paris, 1989.

13. **www.merck.com/mmhe/sec02/ch019/ch019a.html**.

Chapter 3

Natural Healing is Cheap

Oh, that natural stuff is too expensive!

I don't know how many times, as a natural health care practitioner, I've heard words to that effect from potential clients. They think natural food is expensive, that natural medicine methods are expensive, and that natural *anything* is expensive. Let me give it to you straight: That view is nonsense! Actually, the opposite is closer to the truth – generally speaking **natural healing is cheaper than conventional medicine.** Since you've taken my "health dare," it's now my job to prove it to you, which I will do by discussing the costs of:

- Food

- Hospitalization

- Prescription Drugs

- Overall Healthcare

BIGGEST LIE #4

Before I tell you the fourth biggest lie, I need to remind you of the three biggest lies:

> *I'll love you as much in the morning as I do tonight*

> *The check's in the mail*

> *I'm from the government, and I'm here to help you*

Now, may I submit **Biggest Lie #4**:

> ***My insurance pays for it***

Practically everyone with health insurance thinks their healthcare is free (or mostly free). Nothing could be further from the truth! The fallacious logic is that my conventional medical care doesn't cost me anything because "insurance pays for it," while any natural healing approach I do will cost me out-of-pocket.

First of all, your health insurance is hardly free. No employer "gives" you free health insurance. Your employer is simply paying part of your compensation in terms of health insurance rather than cash. It gives the illusion of being free, but it really isn't. If you were not getting that "free" health insurance, market supply and demand would force your employer to pay you more money. Any way you cut it, your employer is going to devote so much expense to employee compensation, whether it is direct in the form of your paycheck or indirect in the form of health insurance or other so-called "benefits." As the old saying goes, "There ain't no free lunch" or any free health care for that matter.

The concept of employer paid health insurance got going during World War II when there were wage and price controls. Employers couldn't offer higher wages to attract a desirable employee, but they could offer non-wage "benefits" that legally increased the actual compensation. What started as a dodge around stupid wage and price control laws spread, becoming the accepted method of compensation. In reality health insurance is just another shell game where you *think* you have something you really don't have.

INSURANCE IS EXPENSIVE

Not only is health insurance not free – it's downright expensive! The Department of Health and Human Services (HHS) reported on March 31, 2014 that the average cost for a middle tier "Silver" plan under the Affordable Care Act (Obamacare) was $328 per month.[1] Imagine writing out a check for that every month (if you're not already doing so). Understand that price is just for an individual. A whole family can cost $1000 to even $2000 per month. This is almost funny to me because you couldn't spend that much money in a month at my natural health care clinic.

This would encourage the question then of why does health insurance cost so much? Let me share several reasons:

1. The patient is not spending his own money – Therefore, he doesn't care what the doctor's charging. In fact, in most cases he won't even *know* what the doctor's charging. The attitude is simply, "I don't care; insurance is paying for it." On the other end of the transaction, the doctor is similarly off the hook from having to deal dollars and cents with the patient because "insurance will pay for it."

Can you imagine what would happen if other financial transactions in your life were handled by an unrelated third party? What if you had "grocery insurance" and just showed a "grocery card" when you went to the supermarket. There would be no prices on any of the food; you would just get what you need and let your grocery insurance pay for it. What would happen? Think prices would go up? Why not – you neither know nor care what the price is. Think quality would go down? Why not – you've eliminated price competition.

2. Curse of the machines. As about everyone knows, conventional healthcare in America is pretty high tech, with lots of very expensive machines – CT, MRI, PET, DEXA, and a whole alphabet soup. When you have a lot of high tech gadgets, they have to get used to amortize their expense. The result is that tests will often be done without a compelling reason – just because the technology is there. I call it "the curse of the machines." The best health practitioners rely not on the "machines," but on their experience-conditioned intuition. The wisest doctor will have a "sense" of what's wrong with you, in many cases, without a lot of expensive diagnostics. This isn't to say we shouldn't do the expensive diagnostics when they're called for, given they can be life-saving. The point is simply that they're overused, driving up healthcare costs and therefore driving up insurance costs.

MARKETING BY OVER-DIAGNOSIS

Not to sound totally cynical, but most (especially high-tech) diagnostics end up being marketing tools, intentionally or unintentionally. The more detail that a given diagnostic test offers, the more it may show up things of no significant consequence. Mammograms are a perfect example. A woman has a mammogram that shows a small lesion, has surgery and then maybe radiation or chemotherapy – all of which are extremely harmful to the immune system and overall health. The truth is that many women have small, insignificant lumps that often disappear on their own through the body's natural healing mechanisms.

We really need to learn when to intervene and when to leave the body alone to its own healing thing. Conventional interventions that really weren't needed can set you up for more serious problems. Obviously this is a fine line to walk: On the one hand a conventional doctor doesn't want to underdiagnose and thereby contribute to illness or death, but that same doctor may commit that same error by over-diagnosing. More often over-diagnosis is the problem, and that makes healthcare and health insurance more expensive.

HOW I AVOIDED OVER-DIAGNOSIS

To motivate you in another way to take the "health dare" of natural healing, let me give a very personal example to illustrate: After years of normal PSA (Prostate Specific Antigen) blood tests, a couple years ago my numbers started going up. I should point out that the PSA test for men is increasingly debated as to its diagnostic value for detecting prostate cancer, given that other factors may cause an increase. Many doctors no longer use it for routine screening. However, rapid increases in the PSA on subsequent tests (called "PSA Velocity") are considered a potentially ominous indicator. In a fourteen month time period I had a 72% increase in my PSA numbers, from 2.5 to 4.3. Good numbers are below 1.0, and it's considered high above 4.0. An increase of 50% in one year may indicate prostate cancer, and an increase of 75% or more in a year may indicate aggressive prostate cancer.

Given that situation, what would you do? Most people would go to the next step of having a prostate biopsy. But I'm not "most people." With the counsel and cooperation of my natural medicine M.D., along with my own clinic's testing methods, I pursued various natural remedies for prostate inflammation, being fairly convinced I did not have cancer. Then the PSA number went even higher – up to 5.5. Would I flinch and run to conventional medicine, or would I still try to find a natural healing solution?

I chose to contact another natural medicine M.D. I work with for his input and got on an even more aggressive program for a couple months. Then the repeat test came back down to 4.0 – though still borderline high, the first time I had been in the normal range in over two years. My "watchful waiting," coupled with an aggressive natural healing approach appears to be paying off. But most guys would just go get the expensive and potentially dangerous biopsy. Had I done that, I would have found out I didn't have cancer, but look at the expense created. Multiply my example times millions of people and it becomes clear why health insurance and conventional healthcare costs are through the roof.

Giving this example I hasten to add that I am *not* telling you, if you happen to be in a similar situation, to avoid expensive diagnostics. This is a very individual decision, based upon your level of knowledge, input from health professionals you trust, your personal convictions on "risk versus reward," and other factors. I can't make that decision for you, but only share my story to illustrate how over-diagnosis increases costs.

LAWYERS – ENTER "DEFENSIVE MEDICINE"

Through often frivolous lawsuits and class actions, lawyers often make healthcare and health insurance more costly. The resulting litigious climate in America drives some doctors out of business, simply from the inability to pay tens or even hundreds of thousands of dollars in malpractice insurance premiums annually. While there are some genuine malpractice cases that truly need financial judgments, almost everyone (except personal injury lawyers) thinks the situation is out of hand.

How many lawyer ads have you seen on TV just today? I think if I see one more mesothelioma ad I'm going to scream! I would think by now that half the country has filed a lawsuit over that disease. These lawyers work on contingency, at no cost to the plaintiff, garnering 30-50% of the judgment if they win. Because the litigation process is so very costly to pursue, most doctors' malpractice insurance companies settle out of court, essentially yielding to a "shake-down" that regrettably is *less* expensive than going to trial. For every dollar you pay in health insurance costs, a significant part of that dollar is funding this perverse legal system. Tort reform with award limit and "loser pays" would eliminate much of this problem and significantly lower insurance costs.

On the lighter side I must include one token lawyer joke:

> *Lawyers and computers have both been proliferating since 1970. Unfortunately, lawyers, unlike computers, have not gotten twice as smart and half as expensive every 18 months.*

IS NATURAL FOOD EXPENSIVE?

A big part of doing "natural healing" is doing "natural food." Do you think natural food is more expensive than your **S**tandard **A**merican **D**iet (SAD Diet)? Let's compare "natural" food with "junk food" in order to determine which is *really* more expensive. Let's take potatoes for example:

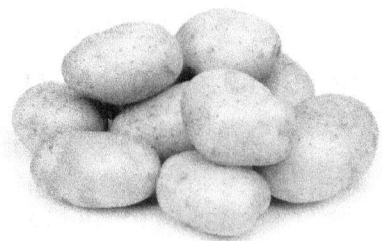

Organically-grown potatoes in this week's Safeway ad cost $1.00 per pound.

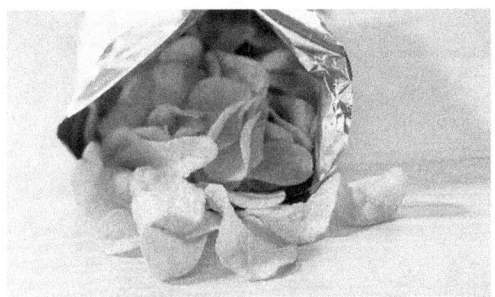

Then we have potato chips – basically a junk food by several criteria. Just 10 ounces of these in the same ad costs $3.50. In other words the natural food version of potatoes cost *less than one-third* what the junk food form does.

How about another example? Lucky Charms refined and highly sugared breakfast cereal at Wal-Mart today costs $3.98 for 20.5 ounces.

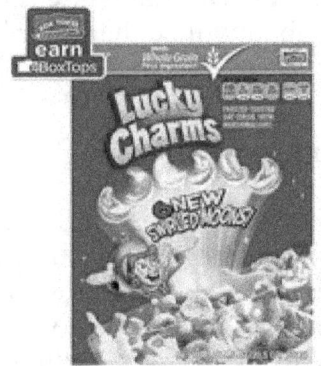

 Meanwhile, more than twice as much Old Fashioned Quaker Oats sells for $2.98.

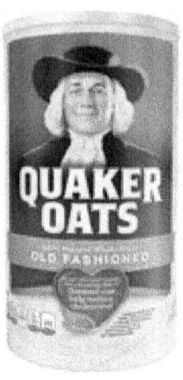

Time and again you will find the less refined, non-sugared product is a much better deal.

Another way of looking at this is comparing cost per nutrient. You get more nutrients in the natural, unrefined foods, so the value is even greater than just comparing ounces to ounces or pounds to pounds. If you're buying **nutritional content** rather than just bulk, empty calories, natural food will be the better buy.

EXPENSIVE OR NOT

Whether natural food is more expensive depends a lot on you. You need to "shop smart." Here's an example: I became interested in using Pomegranate Juice awhile back and was checking out prices. At one national chain natural food store it was over $10 a bottle for a well-known brand, but at another store selling their own private label brand it was about half that cost. You really need to study what things cost at different stores.

ORGANIC PRODUCE

I suspect that most people would include eating organically-grown produce as part of eating a natural food diet. I buy organic produce whenever possible, but am also cost conscious about it. The truth is that some products are more important than others to get organically-grown, due to the wide variance in pesticide residues.

A 2010 study by the Environmental Working Group listed the 12 most and least contaminated produce items. Going "organic" on the most contaminated foods is worth the cost and on the least contaminated is really not worth the cost. Following these guidelines helps make natural food eating less expensive than it otherwise might be.

When Organic is Worth It – 12 Most Contaminated Foods

Grapes

Cherries

Nectarines

Strawberries

Potatoes

Spinach

Blueberries

Peaches

Kale/collard greens

Sweet bell peppers

Apples

Celery

Organic Not Worth It – 12 Least Contaminated Foods

Onions

Pineapple

Asparagus

Eggplant

Avocados

Mango

Kiwi

Cantaloupe

Frozen sweet corn

Frozen sweet peas

Cabbage

Watermelon

BALANCING COST VS. BENEFIT

So how do you process this information on a practical level? On the foods with the highest pesticide residues I *either* buy organic or do without it if the price is too high. On the lowest pesticide residue foods, I generally don't bother with getting organically-grown. This way food costs don't get out of hand. Understand that even if you're paying a bit more, you're also buying a *greater health value* nutritionally and avoiding the health detriment toxin-wise. In this sense many natural foods may in reality be *less* expensive, since in paying more you are also getting more. "Cost" is not always just dollars.

HOSPITALIZATION – YOUR BIGGEST HEALTHCARE COST

When occasionally a potential client, considering my "health dare," thinks my clinic's natural healing program is expensive, I say, "Compared to what?" Let me explain: The first *year* on our Pacific Health Balancing Program (including however many appointments are needed—average is 8) costs about $1000, including the Hand Cradle device that plugs into your computer for remote testing. This would translate to about $125 per one hour testing appointment. The chiropractor I go to charges $45 for a 15 minute appointment – that is, $180 per hour. The holistic MD I go to charges $125 for 20 minutes—that is, $375/hour. The key to honestly evaluating health appointment costs is to look at price per hour, plus the amount of information delivered.

But hospitalization is the really expensive item. On the fairly rare occasions when a client complains about costs, I often reply that our costs are a lot cheaper than a day in the hospital. Here are the statistics:[2]

Average Hospitalization Cost Per Day in 2010

State/Local Government Hospital $1625

Non-Profit Hospital $2025

For-Profit Hospital $1629

Average Hospital Stay Cost in 2010

$9700

Up from $6700 in 1997

Hospital Stay Cost by Illness

Septicemia $18,400

Osteoarthritis $15,100

Acute myocardial infarction (heart attack) $18,200

Respiratory failure $22,300

Complications of surgery or medical care $12,500

Fracture of neck or hip $15,100

So, what do we say about hospitalization? Three things:

1. It is very expensive

2. It is usually the result of *not* preventing illness

3. Natural medicine is the key to prevention and minimizing the need for hospitalization.

NATURAL HEALING VS. PRESCRIPTION DRUG COSTS

Do you still think natural healing is expensive? If so, compared to what? If you think natural healing is expensive, I would simply call your attention to prescription drug prices *as compared to* nutritional supplements. Again I would remind you that the "But my insurance pays for the drugs" line really doesn't cut it – you are ultimately paying for the drugs via wage deferral from your employer, taxes, or directly out of pocket.

I want to look at the cost of six common prescription drugs under the following criteria:

- Cost of taking just *one pill per day* for *one year*

- Comparing the cost on 12/31/10 with the cost on 8/27/14

- Prices are taken from the Costco.com pharmacy website[3]

Here are the numbers:

Lipitor (10 mg) $2164 (up from $1055 on 12/31/10)

Lexapro (5 mg) $2416 (up from $1034)

Nexium (20 mg) $3066 (up from $1964)

Singulair (10 mg) $2510 (up from $1453)

Prevacid (15 mg) $3681 (up from $2143)

Zoloft (50 mg) $2330 (up from $1307)

Understand that the above prices are for just *one* pill or capsule per day of *one* drug – I'm sure many prescriptions are for a higher dosage. On top of that, many people are on several prescription drugs simultaneously. To that point, here are some more statistics:[4]

- 4 billion prescriptions are written each year

- $325 billion was spent on prescriptions in 2012 (3 times as much as 1997)

- 46% of Americans take prescription drugs

- Average number of prescriptions – 4.1 per year

- There are 80 drug ads every hour on American TV

So what do the remedies of natural healing cost by comparison? There are literally tens of thousands of vitamin, mineral, enzyme, herbal, amino acid, and homeopathic products, so I'm speaking very generally. There are also great variations in ingredient quality and avoidance of chemical preservatives, coloring, etc. In my practice we only use "professional line" products – those not sold in stores and only available from health professionals – that are significantly higher quality and therefore more expensive.

Having said that, the average professional-line multi-vitamin we provide costs $20-$30 per month, depending on dosage. Most multi-minerals, digestive enzymes and other categories are in a similar price range. Frankly, we don't even have any products that cost as much as some of the more common prescription drugs that are $75 - $100 or more per bottle. As noted in the previous chapter, virtually no one dies from taking vitamins, while fatal reactions to prescription drugs comprises the fourth leading cause of death in America![5]

TOTAL HEALTHCARE COSTS

Let's get to the big picture of the overall costs of conventional medicine compared to natural healing. The exponential growth of these costs is downright crazy! Take a look at these numbers for overall health care spending in America in dollars and as a percentage of the Gross Domestic Product (GDP):[6]

    1960 $27 billion (5% of the GDP)

    1990 $600 billion (12% of the GDP)

    Today $2.8 trillion (17% of the GDP)

The real question is whether we're getting our money's worth with these astronomical costs. An effective way of measuring this is to look at **conventional medicine per capital cost versus the lifespan produced.** The contrast below shows how ineffective and terribly expensive conventional healthcare in America really is:[7]

    U. S. – 79 years with $8223 (per capita healthcare expense)

Cyprus – 82 years with $2218

Spain – 82 years with $3057

Australia – 83 years with $3685

Japan – 84 years with $3120

How would this compare to natural healing? For $8223 per year you could see a chiropractor every one to two days. You and about ten members of your family could do an annual program at my clinic. The point is simply that a safe, effective, preventive health program could be yours for a fraction of conventional medicine costs. The fact that natural healing is cheap compared to conventional medicine is one of the greatest motivations to take the "health dare."

COST SAVINGS FROM PREVENTION

Natural healing approaches are strongly preventive – that's where they really excel. Prevention automatically leads to saving money in the long-term. Though many medical doctors would wish otherwise, most conventional medicine is not preventive, but more often intervenes after you already have a significant problem, often at the later stages. There is a lot more to be said about the preventive aspect of natural healing, however, which we'll now turn our attention to.

CHAPTER THREE FOOTNOTES

1. http://www.nbcwashington.com/news/health/NATL-ACA-328-Average-Monthly-Health-Insurance-Cost-Under-the-Affordable-Care-Act--225324422.html

2. http://www.beckershospitalreview.com/lists/average-cost-per-inpatient-day-across-50-states-in-2010.html

3. Costco.com pharmacy prices 12/31/09 and 8/27/14

4. "Over Prescribed America at www.topmastersinhealthcare.com/drugged-america/

5. Ibid.

6. Centers for Medicare & Medicaid Services

Chapter 4

Natural Healing is Preventive

Your car versus your body: Which do you take better care of? You first reaction is to probably think:

Of course I take better care of my body!

Let me challenge you. What would you think of someone who:

Never got new tires – they just waited for blow-outs

Never changed the oil – waited for the engine to burn up

Never got a tune-up – just waited until the car wouldn't start

In other words, visualize a person who takes the "If it ain't broke, don't fix it" adage to the extreme.

Of course you would think that someone treating their car that way was a complete moron. How could anyone be that stupid? Don't they know how unsafe and costly that approach is? Don't they know that prevention is cheaper than having to prematurely buy a new car?

Now look in the mirror. You have my permission to call yourself a moron now. We get it when it comes to understanding the implications of not practicing prevention with a car, but that's exactly what we do with our bodies. Rather than maintain (another word for "prevent") we wait for the breakdown and then seek healthcare. But that can change. You can reap the enormous benefits of the health prevention natural healing offers – a great motivation to take the "health dare" of trying natural healing.

"HAVE TO" HEALTHCARE

What's your approach to healthcare? Are you *proactive*, practicing prevention, or *reactive*, waiting until some symptom is manifesting to take action? If you're like most people, you do the latter – what I call **"Have to" Healthcare**. I am simply suggesting an opposite course of action with the question, "Why wait until you're sick?" For example in:

> Conventional Medicine – Why wait until you have a heart attack?
>
> Dentistry – Why wait till your teeth fall out?
>
> Chiropractic – Why wait till you're bent over with pain?
>
> Nutritional Healing – Why wait for deficiencies to produce some pathology?

It's always harder (and more expensive) to deal with an already existing health problem rather than preventing it. Which would you rank better or worse with the following examples?

> Wait till your 50-100 pounds overweight, or correct your weight at 10 pounds over?
>
> Wait until you're diagnosed with diabetes, or prevent by correcting your junk food diet?
>
> Wait until your cholesterol is off the charts, or correct the problem early?
>
> Wait till you're crippled with arthritis, or work on it at the first sign?
>
> Wait till female hormone imbalance is destroying your life, or balance the underlying nutrient deficiencies?
>
> Wait until digestive problems are unbearable, or take enzymes as a preventive?

Many examples could be given, but the point is simply this:

> ***To prevent is to act earlier***

You could prevent instead of waiting to treat the problem. I can think of no better example of this than airplane maintenance. You would never get on a plane if the airline's policy wasn't prevention. Do you know that airlines fix their planes when nothing's wrong? They overhaul or replace jet engines that are still working fine. They replace tires on the landing gears that aren't blown and still have tread. In fact, they do thousands of things, **not** waiting for something to go wrong, but based on a preventive maintenance schedule. They act preemptively to avoid a tragedy. Can you imagine what would happen if they did otherwise – if they waited for an engine to fail *before* replacing it?

By definition, prevention is doing something you don't "have to" do.

WHY "HAVE TO" HEALTHCARE?

It's not hard to make the case for prevention in any area of life, including healthcare. So why do we struggle with this concept? Why is "Have to" healthcare the standard operating procedure for most people? I've come up with four reasons:

1. Most people don't like going to doctors. Though there are some wonderful conventional doctors, I think most people would say that, on average, doctors aren't really that pleasant. Most aren't all that personable or communicative, resulting in most patients feeling they're not really getting answers. I have a lot of personal stories I could tell at this point.

As a child in the 1950's my medical doctor was the woman who delivered me. She was stern, arrogant, haughty to the extreme, and had one answer to about every question – "It's a bug!" Years later I saw a nutritionally-oriented physician that had kind of a fetish over typing his consultation notes into his Mac, rather than writing things down. He kept asking me to slow down in explaining things, since he couldn't type fast enough, and hardly ever looked me straight in the eye. I never went back.

In 1994 I experienced both a compression fracture in my back and my first bitter taste of socialized medicine while vacationing in New Zealand. As part of the process I was sent to an orthopedic surgeon at a larger hospital. He talked to me for a couple minutes saying really nothing helpful or encouraging and sent me downstairs to be fitted for a back brace that turned out to be no help. For that I rode 60 miles in an ambulance! Compounding these negative experiences we have HMO's and the so-called "Affordable Care Act" (Obamacare) that cause patients to be stuck with doctors they don't really like.

After over 30 years in practice as a natural healthcare provider I've heard hundreds of stories from my clients about rude and condescending experiences they've had with their medical doctors. I could literally fill a book with them (if I had written them all down and saved them, anyway). There's an interesting biblical principle that relates here:

Knowledge puffs up, but love builds up. (I Corinthians 8:1b)

The most arrogant people are typically the most educated – those with the most knowledge. The problem is that knowledge isn't the ultimate goal, in that it's rather toxic by itself. The goal is *wisdom*, not knowledge. **Wisdom is knowledge applied with a heaping dose of humility.**

Too many doctors apparently think that "M.D." stands for "Minor Deity" and behave accordingly. This is most often reported to me by my clients who have been berated by their MD for doing some natural healing approach with stupid, uniformed statements like:

I'm the doctor here

You don't need vitamins

You get all the vitamins in the food you eat

If you want to see me, you have to do what I say

And on and on it goes. I tell my clients that they don't work for their doctor, but rather their doctor works for them. Thus, if they are ever abusively treated in any way, there are only two words they need to say:

You're fired!

Beyond the above negatives on going to the doctor, medical procedures are often uncomfortable – I mean where else does someone tell you to take off your clothes and insert fingers or instruments into your body orifices? Finally there is the issue of immediate cost if you have a co-pay on health insurance or if a high deductible policy means you're paying it all. All things considered, going to a conventional medical doctor can be a pretty negative experience, so many just don't. This all-too-frequent experience in dealing with conventional doctors should be enough to motivate taking the health dare of natural healing alternatives.

2. The conventional medical system encourages "have to" healthcare.

I see conventional medicine as rather conflicted. On the one hand, emphasis on "preventive care" is kind of the "in thing" with many M.D.'s – more on this later. But, on the other hand, the "system" they practice within is strongly oriented around treatment of existing problems that are often somewhat advanced. Very often a patient with a suspected or minor problem is told the doctor can do nothing *yet* and to "come back when it gets worse." In other words, the doctor wants a symptom *substantial enough to* treat. That certainly rules out prevention, doesn't it!

Then think about typical diagnostic tests, say an X-ray, for example. That diagnostic reveals an abnormality already present and at least somewhat advanced. Your X-ray will never show what *might* happen down the road. Thus, conventional medicine treatments focus on existing, usually well-defined problems that are well beyond the opportunity for prevention.

3. Symptom treating is tied to "have to" healthcare.

Treating symptoms is clearly the focus of conventional medicine. Let me again make this rather obvious point clear: If you're treating symptoms, you are by definition not preventive. A true preventive approach to health care therefore cannot be focused on symptoms, but rather on what is going on *before the symptoms manifest*. As long as conventional medicine continues its focus on "treating disease" (i. e. symptoms) rather than building health, it won't be preventive.

4. Most people have never practiced prevention. As with the oft-repeated words of the Pogo cartoon character, "We have met the enemy, and it is us." Most of us don't think in terms of preventing future health issues, plus we certainly don't act in a preventive way either. Our entire experience with healthcare has largely been with symptom-oriented treatment, rather than root cause prevention. To get the amazing benefits prevention offers, a new philosophy of healthcare must be embraced.

NATURAL HEALING IS LARGELY PREVENTIVE

Though I have emphasized the *preventive* aspect of natural healing, that is not to say that natural remedies don't also correct *existing problems*. For example, natural remedies can be very effective at:

Lowering cholesterol

Lowering blood pressure

Eliminating headaches

Lifting your depression

Reducing or eliminating arthritis or fibromyalgia pain

Resolving your PMS or menopausal symptoms

Correcting various types of digestive distress

Natural healing is almost automatically preventive in its effect, though *in addition* it also often helps existing health symptoms. Because natural healing usually takes more time, one usually doesn't wait for the symptoms to progress. When you start using natural remedies, you tend to be looking for things to "nip in the bud," so to speak.

Lots of research over many decades confirms the preventive value of natural healing. Even many (if not most) in conventional medicine will admit the preventive value of:

- Fiber for colon issues and lowering cholesterol

- Fish oil for cardiovascular health

- Vitamin C for infection prevention

- Echinacea and other herbs for infections

Many specific studies document these and other natural approaches for both their preventive and treatment value.

A fascinating aspect of natural healing involves its effect on multiple fronts. Unlike most drugs, natural remedies are not restricted to a single problem, but rather cross over into other issues as a preventive. Let me give a couple examples. Let's say you're taking a fiber supplement for bowel cleansing and regularity. Though it greatly helps the bowel, it also may have value in lowering cholesterol and reducing allergic sensitivities.

How about taking a fish oil supplement for high cholesterol. The fish oil isn't good *only* for cholesterol lowering, but can help a whole range of other problems – arthritic joint issues, skin health, and memory issues. While taking the natural remedy for a *current* problem, you may also be helping prevent another problem.

CONVENTIONAL "PREVENTIVE HEALTHCARE"

We hear a lot from conventional medicine about "preventive healthcare," but what does that really mean? Everyone (and every health practitioner) has a philosophy of health from which they operate. That philosophy defines the enemy to be defeated, which in turn defines the treatment approach. So what is the enemy? Is the enemy the symptom or the underlying cause?

For example, a conventional doctor typically considers high cholesterol – a symptom -- as the enemy and therefore prescribes a statin drug as the remedy – all in the name of "preventive healthcare." The doctor's philosophy says that high cholesterol causes heart disease (a claim increasingly challenged by natural healing practitioners) and therefore taking a drug to lower cholesterol is deemed "preventive healthcare." Problem is the statin drug has side-effects that produce other health problems, partly due to its inhibition of Co-Enzyme Q10 production – ironically, an essential ingredient for heart health. Can something really be considered good "preventive healthcare" if it causes other health problems?

But that's not all. The high cholesterol is a symptom, not a root cause. So what's causing the high cholesterol? Conventional doctors don't ask that question because their philosophy dictates that the cholesterol symptom **is** the problem. End of story – take this drug. Again I would ask if we really can call an approach "preventive healthcare" when it's only dealing with symptoms while leaving the root cause untouched?

Here's another way of thinking about this: Is your cholesterol high because of a "deficiency" of statin drug? Is your cholesterol high *because* you lack that drug? Of course not! The drug is simply designed to manipulate the cholesterol level, that is, to treat the symptom.

True preventive health care would ask *why* the cholesterol is high. Contrary to the myths perpetuated by the low cholesterol food industry, it's not your eggs, butter, and beef. Cholesterol, among other things, is a repair substance for the blood vessels. Nutrient deficiencies cause the "potholes" in the blood vessels that cholesterol must "patch." Thus, the worse your blood vessels are, the more cholesterol your body **needs** to try to keep you alive. (For a further explanation of the importance of cholesterol and what causes its elevation, see my *Better Health Update* "Cholesterol Confusion" at **www.pacifichealthcenter.com**.)

Examples could be given of what I would call "pseudo-preventive healthcare." One of the most notorious is mammograms for routine breast cancer screening. The documented truth from studies about routine screening mammograms is that:

- They fail to detect 40% of the actual breast cancer

- The radiation itself is carcinogenic

- They don't improve chances of survival

- They find a lot of false positives, resulting in unnecessary and often harmful treatment

(For details on these issues with mammograms, see my *Better Health Update* "Mammograms: Yes or No" at **www.pacifichealthcenter.com**. Again, this represents another example of "pseudo-preventive healthcare rather than true prevention. By contrast a natural healing approach would be especially concerned with nutritional and toxin factors that would predispose a woman to breast cancer such as environmental chemicals with estrogenic mimicking properties – chemicals that can both be avoided and be detoxified from the body.

Natural healing typically views multiple causes that are really at the root of the problem, such as allergic sensitivity, nutrient deficiency, toxins, and others. If you take your focus off of symptoms, instead assessing the body for underlying issues and correcting those, you're actually practicing prevention. Instead of just trying to get a symptom to go away, you're actually trying to build health and balance in the body so that the next symptom never happens. We must understand the real philosophy driving our healthcare decisions (or our doctor's healthcare decisions).Then we can chart a new course. We need a comprehensive view of the health of our bodies – a view that the "health dare" of trying natural healing abundantly offers.

Chapter 5

Natural Healing is Comprehensive

Remember back in elementary school when they talked about health? I remember getting this standard definition:

Health is the absence of disease

So, if I don't have any medically diagnosed diseases, I'm healthy? Are you kidding? How can you *define* something by what it is *not*? Wouldn't it be absurd to say?

A horse is not a cow?

A chair is not a table?

A Ford is not a Chevy or Chrysler?

Telling you what something is **not** doesn't tell you much. If we're going to achieve health, we better know what it actually *is*. Accepting this false view of health leads to employing false treatments that do nothing to resolve your real problems. Enter conventional medicine . . .

CONVENTIONAL MEDICINE VIEW

Just like that grade school health class, conventional medicine largely views health as the absence of disease. Therefore, if you have no symptoms, you're presumed healthy. This flows from the conventional medicine philosophy of **treating symptoms** which follows this formula:

Come to the doctor with a symptom

Get a drug to treat your symptom

If the symptom then goes away, you're healthy

May I illustrate the absurdity of this approach by being absurd? Suppose you have an overflowing toilet causing you to call a plumber. What if the plumber just brought a bunch of towels to soak up the water flowing out from under the bathroom door and gave you a can of air freshener to spray? He would have treated the symptom, but left the root problem intact. You would never accept that "solution" from your plumber, but you accept that solution nearly every time you see your medical doctor. Your body is that overflowing toilet. It is overflowing because it is plugged up and not draining properly. The drugs you're given only spray air freshener on the symptoms leaving the root cause intact.

So what actually happens when you see your doctor? If you have:

High cholesterol – take this drug to lower it

High blood pressure – take this drug to lower it

Depressed – take this drug to manipulate your serotonin levels

Headache – take this drug to make you not feel the headache

So what then is the fallacy? You *don't* have:

High cholesterol because of a *deficiency* of statins

High blood pressure because of a *deficiency* of Lisinopril

Depression because of a *deficiency* of Prozac

Headache because of a *deficiency* of aspirin

Do you see that all this is about one's *philosophy* of healing? My "health dare" to try natural healing is largely directed at those fed up with the false philosophy of much of conventional medicine. There is a better way – a better philosophy of health.

NATURAL HEALING VIEW

Natural healing defines health in a comprehensive way. Though many specific definitions might be used, I like to go back to the etymology of the word health. "Health" comes from the Old English word "hale," which means "whole." Health is therefore about *wholeness*. But wholeness is more than mere *physical* wholeness, since we must look at the total person – body, mind and spirit. If you are whole in body, mind and spirit, you are truly healthy. If you have "holes" in your "wholeness," you are not healthy – it's really that simple. (For a more extensive discussion of wholeness in body, mind and spirit, see my book, *Body, Mind & Health*, linked at the end of this book.)

Natural healing focuses on **root causes**. The issue is not what will make your cholesterol go down, but rather what's causing it to be high in the first place? Everything your body does is for a reason – ultimately for its survival. Samuel Hahnemann, founder of homeopathic medicine put it this way:

> *The symptom is a healing gesture.*

So, start thinking in terms of why does the body *need* high cholesterol. Contrary to the propaganda from the conventional medical drug establishment, cholesterol is an essential nutrient from which your body makes hormones and neurotransmitters. It's also kind of a cardiovascular "spackle" for patching up your blood vessels. If your body "needs" higher cholesterol, it may be because your blood vessels are full of "potholes" needing smoothing over. By the way that poor condition of your blood vessels necessitating the higher cholesterol is related to B-vitamin and other deficiencies. It makes a huge difference in how you approach your health problems when you simply keep tracing them back to root causes.

What about depression? Does it just happen for no reason? Of course not! There are underlying causes that may be physical, mental or spiritual. It's therefore important to discern which area or areas you lack wholeness to determine root causes.

A distinction must be made, however, at this point. Conventional medicine will typically say you have a "chemical imbalance" in your brain causing the depression, such as not enough serotonin neurotransmitter. That may sound like they are dealing with a root cause, but not so. Conventional medicine will stop at this point reasoning, "You have a chemical imbalance of serotonin, so we'll give you a drug to increase the serotonin level." The problem is that they didn't ask the next question:

*What's **causing** the chemical imbalance?*

Pursuing that question will typically lead you to a valid root cause such as a nutrient deficiency.

But what about headaches? Let me ask this first: Do you really just want your headache to go away without dealing with the cause? While you may say, "Yes," if that headache is excruciating right now, is that not an invitation for a greater problem in the future? Do you really want to "cover up" the symptom rather than find the root cause? Think of these illustrations:

Disconnecting that irritating warning light on your dashboard

Taking the battery out of your smoke detector so it stops making noise

Putting a penny behind a fuse that keeps blowing from an overload

There are very negative implications to making a "symptom" go away *without* correcting the underlying *cause* of that symptom.

DISEASE MANAGEMENT VS. DISEASE RESOLUTION

The focus of conventional medicine is, unfortunately, not on solving diseases so much as it is on *managing* them. Conventional medicine doesn't solve your high cholesterol problem, but just manages it with drugs. The same is true for your high blood pressure, arthritis, skin problems, digestive problems, endocrine issues, etc. – you keep the problem and just manage it with drugs. Now I wonder why?

Given the pharmaceutical industry is heavily involved in funding both initial and continuing education of doctors, wouldn't it make sense that the "philosophy" conveyed would tilt toward keeping people on drugs *forever* to manage their symptoms, rather than actually **getting rid of the problem**? There's not much money in curing health problems, but there's a huge residual income to be derived from keeping someone on several $100 a month drugs *the rest of their life*!

Natural healing, as I have been saying, seeks resolution through dealing with the root causes of your health problems. Instead of taking a drug to "manage" the problems for the rest of your life, why not just fix the problem? But here's the rub: If you don't know the root cause, you can't fix it. Conventional medicine typically doesn't even look for that underlying cause, but prefers to stop at the quick fix of the prescription to "manage" it. For most common health problems no diagnostics will be pursued in an attempt to discover a root cause, since that takes more time and money than that system cares to expend. By contrast, natural healing *begins* with assessments oriented around identifying root causes. So, what are these root causes and how do we identify them?

3 BASIC ROOT CAUSES

Fortunately there aren't all that many root causes; in fact, I focus on just three root causes of most health problems. It is my simple thesis that if you identify and resolve these three root causes, these three "common denominators," you will help or eliminate most health problems. Remove these three root causes and you remove the "roadblocks" freeing up your body to heal as God designed. Let's examine them in some detail:

Root Cause #1 – Nutrient Deficiency

Your body is, at least in a sense, a "machine," and a highly complex one at that. As such, machines need fuel to operate. Your body's "fuel" is food, but not just any old food. Your food-fuel must be nutrient-rich in order to supply the vitamins, minerals, amino acids, and enzymes required for healthy function.

Enter the "Big Lie" that countless people have heard from their medical doctor:

You get all the vitamins you need in the food you eat

Doctors who make that rather ridiculous statement must also be omniscient, since they must know just what kind of food you are eating to make such a pronouncement! Would they really say you're getting all the vitamins you need from the food you eat if you are living on fast food or candy bars? Or perhaps they believe in some sort of alchemy where, instead of turning lead into gold, they believe your digestive tract can magically turn junk food into healthy, nutrient-rich food.

This really isn't rocket science to understand. Take any food crop as an example. Most commercial foods are grown with synthetic fertilizer – NPK – nitrogen, phosphorus, and potash, a mere three minerals being replaced from those depleted in the soil. But what about the other 80+ minerals *not* replaced with synthetic fertilizer? Those minerals would be present in organically grown crops grown with natural fertilizers. Through synthetic agriculture we have spent decades "mining" the soil instead of farming it. Is it any wonder the foods, though large and pretty, lack so many nutrients? Most people live on **foodless food**.

But do the numbers really back this assertion? What is the extent of nutrient deficiencies in America? Here are the numbers according to the *Journal of Nutrition*:[1]

25% are deficient in Vitamin C

34% are deficient in Vitamin A

38% are deficient in Calcium

45% are deficient in Magnesium

60% are deficient in Vitamin E

70% are deficient in Vitamin D

Too many people (and doctors) equate a full stomach with good nutrition. You can fill your stomach with all kinds of good tasting junk, yet, nutritionally speaking, be starving to death, and thus produce all manner of health problems.

So what happens when you are nutrient deficient? First of all, your body cannot function *optimally*. This would be like running your car on watered-down gasoline: Initially it will produce poor performance, while eventually it will cause a breakdown. That "breakdown," when we're talking about your body is called disease.

Root Cause #2 – Food & Environmental Sensitivity

So what is a food or environmental sensitivity? Though it may seem like just semantics, we must distinguish between "sensitivity" and "allergy." Allergy is a conventional medical term for a significant immune system reaction to a substance, usually measured either in the blood or on the skin. Symptoms like rashes and hives and even anaphylactic shock might be manifested with such an allergic reaction. A relatively small percentage of the population has true medical allergies.

By contrast *sensitivity* refers to more of a *digestive*, rather than an immune system reaction to a substance. Essentially the term "sensitivity" refers to any way someone is adversely affected by contact with a particular food or environmental item. Unlike medical allergies, about everyone has food, and usually environmental, sensitivities – it's just a question of how many and how severe.

Incomplete digestion results in food components that *should* have been absorbed in the upper digestive tract ending up in the lower digestive tract where they don't belong. That sets off some alarms resulting in the sensitivity symptoms – digestive reactions, fatigue, mood changes, or many other possibilities. Authorities indicate that well over 100 common symptoms *can be* caused by food sensitivities.

But what about environmental sensitivities to things like dust, pollen, animal dander, and mold? Food sensitivities are really the key to the environmental reactions in that you first have food sensitivities with the environmental sensitivities developing as a result. In my own practice of over 30 years I've found that the environmental sensitivities typically improve with the correction of the food sensitivities.

The real question concerns how we can correct the food and environmental sensitivities and thus remove this "common denominator" of many health problems. Here are the steps I follow in my practice:

1. Improve the digestion with digestive enzymes. Most people are deficient in hydrochloric acid and enzymes after age 40 or even earlier. Since inadequate digestion is the root cause of sensitivities, we must start here.

2. Repair the digestive tract. Years of eating the wrong foods in the wrong way often damages the mucosal surfaces of the intestines. This may result in problems like Leaky Gut Syndrome, colitis, diverticulitis, Irritable Bowel Syndrome, and other digestive ailments. Various herbal, fiber, amino acid, and other remedies can help in the repair.

3. Re-implant beneficial bacteria. Unfortunately the average person has taken in loads of antibiotic drugs, if not as actual prescriptions, through eating meat from animals given antibiotics. Your digestive tract needs the beneficial acidophilus and other organisms to function optimally. Probiotic supplements will successfully replace these absent organisms.

4. Homeopathic desensitizing. Homeopathic remedies for food and environmental sensitivities involve micro-dilutions of the sensitive substances taken as drops under the tongue. The homeopathic food or environmental remedy, though not the substance itself, is recognized by the body and associated with that sensitive item. Essentially the homeopathic remedy is nothing but an energetic imprint of the item – sort of like looking at a picture of an apple versus taking a bite out of one. The homeopathic remedy thus presents a reminder to the body of that food or environmental substance in a non-threatening way that requires no reaction. As with the apple, the body recognizes the "picture," but doesn't react to actually eating it. By taking the remedy for a few weeks the body is reconditioned to not react, desensitizing it to that item. Homeopathic desensitizing is the most specific and effective method I have found for dealing with this root cause of many health problems.

Root Cause #3 – Toxins

Of these three "common denominator" causes of health problems, I believe toxins are the most significant. So what are we talking about when we refer to "toxins?" Here's a list of categories of common toxins:[2]

Industrial chemicals

Pesticides

Food additives

Dead bacteria or viruses

Medical drugs

Hydrocarbon-based chemicals

Heavy metals

So, how do we get toxic? How about the air you breathe and the water you drink? Many of these toxins are literally everywhere, such that it's hard *not* to be exposed. Specifically we have the issue of chemical toxins. I would note that there are 84,000 chemicals legal for commerce in the United States – a 25-fold increase since World War II. Cosmetics use 13,000 chemicals, with only 10% of those having been evaluated for safety.[3] That's a lot of possible toxin exposure.

One of the most disturbing aspects of chemical toxicity is the property many chemicals have for mimicking hormones, the imbalance of which can lead to cancer. For example, the Silent Spring Institute tested 120 homes in 2004 for 89 endocrine disrupting chemicals. In these 120 homes they discovered 67 of the 89 chemicals were present. In addition, they found two-thirds of the homes tested positive for DDT though it was banned from usage 40 years ago![4]

What about some of the other categories of toxins? Prescription drugs represent a significant toxicity to the body. Understand that even the most helpful and appropriately prescribed drug is foreign to the body. When you put something into your body that isn't good food, your body will treat that substance as a toxin. It will then either try to eliminate it through the various elimination pathways, or if it can't eliminate it, store it somewhere out of the way, usually in fatty tissue. Every drug you take creates an additional elimination burden on the body.

The last category in the above list is heavy metals. This includes mercury, lead, aluminum, nickel, cadmium, arsenic and various other toxins. Like the chemical category, these substances are common in the overall environment through air, water, and other physical contact. But perhaps the most significant heavy metal toxin is dental mercury, as found in amalgam dental fillings.

So-called "silver fillings" are actually about 50% mercury and 30% silver. One hundred million Americans have amalgam fillings in their mouths. Mercury amalgam fillings have been around for about 150 years, though they were hotly debated as to safety in their early days in the nineteenth century. In fact, the American Dental Association was started specifically to promote mercury amalgams over an opposing dental association.

The dental establishment position over all these years was that mercury didn't escape from the amalgam filling once it was mixed and placed in the mouth. Modern laboratory techniques, such as mercury vapor analyzers however, have now clearly shown that mercury vapor is continuously emitted from the fillings, especially in an acidic, warm environment – like when you drink a cup of hot coffee.

Mercury is the second most toxic element on the Periodic Table, second only to plutonium. A holistic dentist friend of mine jokes that conventional dentistry would probably make fillings out plutonium if they could! Though still endorsed as safe by the American Dental Association, more and more dentists are quietly switching to composite fillings (space-age plastics) usually citing "cosmetic" reasons. The reality, of course, is that common sense is dictating that putting such a highly toxic material in your mouth just can't be safe. The Environmental Protection Agency (EPA) has stringent rules for the disposal of dental mercury and major fines for violations. Mercury is considered toxic before it's put in your mouth and after it's removed. In the conventional dentistry view apparently the only safe place for mercury is in your mouth! I only wish they were kidding.

SELF-PRODUCED TOXICITY

There are just two ways of getting toxic: You can either take toxins into your body from the outside, as we've been discussing, or you can **make your own toxins** inside your body. As bad as the chemicals, heavy metals, and others that enter from the outside, the internally, self-produced toxins are probably worse. This again goes back to digestion with my **Number One Rule of Health**:

> *Anything you eat that you don't fully digest, assimilate and eliminate becomes a toxin.*

Imagine that! You have your own little "toxin factory" in your digestive tract when it's not working properly. It's really not an overstatement to say that, "Digestion is everything" when it comes to health. Optimizing your digestion will do wonders for lowering your overall toxicity.

DEALING WITH TOXICITY

Resolving toxicity (not "managing" it) is relatively simple with just two steps:

1. Stop the toxic input. Think of your body as a bathtub with a faucet for putting in water and a drain for letting it out. But let's suppose that the faucet is not adding pure water to the tub, but all manner of toxins. The obvious first step to detoxification would be to turn off that faucet, stopping the toxic input. No matter how efficiently the drain is getting rid of those toxins, as long as you keep adding more your body will be toxic. Unfortunately, many people are adding toxins at a much greater rate than their bodies can eliminate them, so merely stopping the toxic input isn't enough – you have to get rid of the toxins already present.

2. Stimulate detoxification. A number of options are available to detoxify the body. Keep in mind that your body was created to naturally detoxify, and it constantly does just that through the liver, kidneys, bowel, lungs, skin, and other elimination pathways. Our purpose is not to do something the body is not doing, but rather to **augment the body's natural detoxification** processes to get the best results. Different detoxification methods will be more appropriate or more available depending on the person and the health problems involved:

> **Cleansing Diets** – Generally a cleansing diet will focus on some combination of fruits and vegetables, leaving off starches and meat. Though there are many different versions of this approach, I often recommend our **7-Day Cleansing Diet**, which is available at the following link:
> http://www.pacifichealthcenter.com/blog/?page_id=152

> **Fasting** – There are essentially two types of fasting: Juice fasting, which is more like the cleansing diet above or plain water fasting – sometimes called a "normal fast" – where only water is consumed. Juice fasting utilizes the cleansing effect of the fruit or vegetable juices used, while normal water fasting causes the body to "live off itself" by burning up unnecessary junk, particularly fat that is storing a lot of toxins. Most juice fasts or normal water fasts are done for one to three days, though it is possible to go longer, depending on the individual and the problems being addressed.

> **Dry Infrared Sauna** – Saunas have been around for centuries as a method of sweating out toxins through the skin. Modern dry infrared saunas are even more effective than the traditional

saunas. Given the investment in purchasing the sauna, this method is not as common, though its adherents swear by it.

Exercise – Just plain old exercise is one of the greatest ways to stimulate detoxification. Increased circulation and perspiration enhance the removal of toxins.

Homeopathic Detoxification. The most specific method of detoxification utilizes homeopathic medicine. This utilizes a homeopathic micro-dilution of a given toxin, such as mercury, for example. While consuming mercury makes you mercury toxic, the homeopathic dilution of mercury does just the opposite, stimulating the detoxification of that element. The homeopathic remedy is like a "wanted poster" placed where all the immune system "bounty hunters" will read it, attuning them to what "outlaw" to go after and destroy. There are both general homeopathic remedies for *categories* of toxins, such as chemicals or heavy metals, as well as individual remedies that can be made up for specific toxins based on testing.

CONCLUSION

A monumental difference exists between conventional medicine and natural healing. I have focused on the term **comprehensive** to describe that difference. Most conventional medicine operates on the surface level – identifying symptoms and then prescribing drugs to modify those symptoms. Most doctors seldom probe deeper to discover the underlying root causes, since it's a lot easier to just push pills for fixing symptoms.

The problem is that nothing really gets fixed, but only managed until a premature death. Nowhere is this huge difference in the approach to healthcare better explained than in a humorous, yet serious tract called, *The American Death Ceremony* (author unknown) that may nudge you a little more toward the health dare of trying natural healing:

> *The death ceremony started as a crude ritual back in the days of witchcraft. In recent years it has been developed into a science. It usually takes from 10 to 15 years, however modern advancements are shortening this period of time.*

It starts with a simple aspirin for a simple headache. When one aspirin will no longer cover up the headache, take two. After a few months, when two aspirins will no longer cover up the headache, you take one of the stronger compounds. By this time it becomes necessary to take something for the ulcers that have been caused by the aspirin.

Now that you are taking two medicines, you have a good start. After a few months, these medicines will disrupt your liver function. If a good infection develops, you can take some penicillin. Of course the penicillin will damage your red blood corpuscles and spleen so that you develop anemia.

By this time all these medications will put such a strain on your kidneys they should break down. It is now time to take some antibiotics. When these destroy your natural resistance to disease, you can expect a general flair-up of all your symptoms. The next step is to cover up all of these symptoms with sulfa drugs.

When the kidneys finally plug up you can have them drained. Some poisons will build up in your system, but you can keep going quite a while this way. By now the medications will be so confused they won't know what they are supposed to be doing, but it really doesn't matter. If you have followed every step as directed you can now make an appointment with your undertaker.

This game is played by almost all Americans.

CHAPTER 5 FOOTNOTES

1. *Journal of Nutrition*, August 2011

2. Kenyon, Julian, *21st Century Medicine*

3. http://articles.mercola.com/sites/articles/archive/2014/10/25/dangers-everyday-industrial-chemicals.aspx

4. http://www.silentspring.org/breast-cancer-and-environment/fact-sheets

Chapter 6

Natural Healing is Complementary

Are you struggling with this question:

> *If I go "natural" does that mean I leave conventional medicine altogether?*

That's kind of a scary thought, isn't it? It's an issue you probably want to resolve before taking my natural healing "health dare." After all, we've relied on conventional medicine our whole lives, and frankly we all know conventional medicine is good, at least for some things. Well, the short answer to the above question is an emphatic **"No."** Natural healing does not demand exclusivity – you don't have to burn all your conventional medicine bridges behind you. Natural healing can often (but not 100% of the time) be used *in conjunction with* conventional medicine. Let's unpack this and see how it works.

WHAT DOES "COMPLEMENTARY" MEAN?

Note that we are talking about "complementary" with an "e," not "complimentary" with an "i." This isn't about telling you how nice you look, but about how two things together can enhance a result. The basic dictionary definition of "complementary" in our usage is:

> *Making up what is lacking in another*

"Complementary" medicine assumes that both conventional and natural healing methods can often work together to bring about a better result. However, this does raise two issues:

1. Conventional medicine can compete with natural healing and negate results.

2. However, conventional medicine may be necessary to control symptoms, and thus must be done.

CONVENTIONAL MEDICINE IS NEEDED

By extolling the virtues of natural healing I am in no way saying you should throw out conventional medicine. Though I do believe that conventional medicine is used too much overall, it is needed for the following:

1. Diagnostics – Conventional medicine offers some amazing diagnostic capabilities *if you really need them*. There is a time for X-rays, CT scans, MRI's, etc. But these can also be overused. It's important to wisely discern what is really needed versus:

> Diagnostics just being used because they're available (as in "Never ask a barber if you need a haircut")

> Diagnostics being used for defensive medicine (what might be called "CYA" medicine)

2. Acute emergency situations—We need conventional medicine for accidents, burns, lacerations, broken bones, and other acute or emergency events. Conventional medicine excels in this area.

3. Advanced problems too late for natural healing – I can give a personal example here. I take two prescription drugs for an adrenal condition that has no natural healing alternative. BUT, I also do lots of natural healing as a complementary approach, including remedies to help negate side-effects from those prescription drugs. Unfortunately there are some health conditions that are beyond healing and can only be managed.

Beyond the above three exceptions, natural healing can usually complement conventional medicine. However, most are unaware of their alternatives, falsely assuming that straight conventional medicine is the only option. Such a view is unfortunately encouraged by conventional medicine, as a little history will demonstrate.

CONVENTIONAL MEDICINE'S WAR WITH CHIROPRACTIC

For decades conventional medicine belittled and undermined chiropractic until five chiropractors got fed up. In 1976 Chester Wilks and four other chiropractors sued the American Medical Association for violating the Sherman Anti-Trust Act. After failing to gain relief in their original suit, a second suit was successful in 1987. The court ruled that the AMA had indeed engaged in an unlawful conspiracy against chiropractic. Up until 1983 the AMA had labeled chiropractic an "unscientific cult" and held it unethical for MD's to associate with chiropractors.[1] Beyond the legal aspects involved, this case simply reflected the *exclusivity* that conventional medicine has historically demanded. In effect MD's were the "union members" and all other health practitioners were the "scabs" needing to be eliminated. The increasingly popular view of *complementary* medicine is fortunately changing that.

AMA WAR WITH HOMEOPATHY

Undermining chiropractic wasn't the AMA's first foray into conspiring against other healing approaches, though. They nearly destroyed homeopathy. The American Institute of Homeopathy was founded in 1844. Two years later the AMA was founded, largely to suppress homeopathic medicine. In 1900 20% of the MD's in America were homeopaths. At that time there were 22 homeopathic medical schools and over 100 homeopathic hospitals. Homeopathy was a wildly successful healing approach whose results far surpassed conventional medicine (allopathy) in dealing with the 1918 flu epidemic. Homeopathy had gained strong supporters including John D. Rockefeller, William James, Louisa May Alcott, Harriet Beecher Stowe, Samuel Morse, and Henry Wadsworth Longfellow.

Then the conspiracy began. First, the AMA expelled homeopathic doctors from their "approved" societies. Then the AMA Code of Ethics forbade consulting with homeopathic MD's. These restrictions resulted in declining enrollments at homeopathic medical schools, which then either closed down or converted to allopathic, drug-oriented conventional medicine.

Homeopathy largely became extinct in America in the first half of the 20th century, only surviving because of its continued popularity in Europe, India and elsewhere. Homeopathy is thriving today, in part due to two states – Nevada and Arizona – that license Homeopathic Medical Doctors through a separate licensing board.

CONDITIONS RESPONDING TO NATURAL HEALING

So where does natural healing really work best? Is it applicable to *any* healing situation or just to some? When should conventional medicine be embraced, and when should it be avoided? Here are a few guidelines:

1. Conventional medicine is most appropriate for acute, traumatic situations. This isn't really rocket science. If you break your arm, if you have a laceration, if you're in a car accident, if you're severely burned, rely on conventional medicine. It truly shines in these areas. Think about it: If you have a compound fracture with bloody bones protruding, do you really want to go to some holistic doctor that asks you, "How's the stress in your life lately?" **With acute situations treating the symptom makes sense.**

2. Natural healing is usually the most appropriate for chronic, non-life threatening health problems. Conventional medicine's focus on symptom treatment fails with most chronic problems. This false philosophy of healing inevitably fails, leaving the victim at best dependent on symptom-treating drugs. Chronic conditions require identifying and resolving root causes. Natural healing excels in these areas.

3. Natural healing can *usually* provide complementary benefits to required conventional treatment. As is the point of this chapter, conventional medicine and natural healing need not necessarily be exclusive, but rather can work together. Going back to the broken arm illustration, proper nutritional supplementation will enhance healing. Natural anti-inflammatories can reduce pain and swelling, potentially lessening the need for side-effect producing drugs.

Let's look at some common health problems that usually respond very well to natural healing.

COLDS & SINUS INFECTIONS

This is very possibly the most common health problem. The typical conventional medicine approach with over the counter or prescription drugs is often pointless. Colds are viral infections, as are most sinus infections. Yet, antibiotics drugs are very commonly prescribed to the sufferers. That may fill a psychological need in the patient with a "Doctor, please do something!" mentality, but it is no real value. The dirty little secret is that antibiotics *only* kill bacteria and are therefore of no value against viral infections. Though every MD knows this, they nevertheless give out antibiotic prescriptions by the millions for those afflicted with colds and sinus infections. This isn't just a waste of money on prescriptions, but something far worse. Overuse of antibiotics causes *Candida* yeast overgrowth, increased antibiotic resistance, and depression of future immunity.

This prevalent misuse of antibiotics prompted the Centers for Disease Control (CDC) to start a campaign a few years ago called **"Snort, Sniffle, Sneeze. No Antibiotics Please!"** The following is taken from the CDC's website:

> *Are you aware that colds, flu, most sore throats, and bronchitis are caused by viruses? Did you know that antibiotics do not help fight viruses? It's true. Plus, taking antibiotics when you have a virus may do more harm than good. Taking antibiotics when they are not needed increases you risk of getting an infection later that resists antibiotic treatment.* [2]

The Mayo Clinic has issued a similar warning, noting which infections are bacterial and which are viral:

> *Antibiotics are effective against bacterial infections, certain fungal infections and some kinds of parasites. Antibiotics don't work against viruses.*

Their article goes on to list the following infections that are bacterial and therefore may be helped by antibiotics: bladder infections, wound and skin infections such as staph, severe sinus infections lasting longer than two weeks, some ear infections, and strep throat. Then they list viral infections *not* helped by antibiotics: bronchitis, colds flu, most coughs, most ear infections, most sore throats, and stomach flu.[3]

"SELECTIVE BREEDING" OF BACTERIA

I've often told my seminar audiences that taking antibiotics can comprise a "selective breeding" program to make stronger and more resistant bacteria. Here's the logic: When you take that antibiotic prescription do you think that drug kills 100% of the bacteria in your body? Probably not. Well then, which bacteria do you think survive the antibiotic drug assault? Wouldn't it be the really strong and tough ones – you know, the bacteria with black leather jackets and tattoos riding around on big motorcycles? So the antibiotic killed off the weaker "wimpy" bacteria – got them easily – but it didn't eradicate the really tough bacteria **that live to reproduce themselves.** So what are you really doing when you take an antibiotic but practicing a **selective breeding program to make stronger bacteria!** Thus we create "super germs" that no antibiotic drug will kill.

So what about natural approaches to dealing with colds and sinus infections? Natural healing offers a very different approach. Instead of trying to kill germs with the outside agent of drugs, it instead seeks to build up the immune system. Natural healing recognizes that the most powerful healing comes, not from drugs, but from the constantly operating immune system God created.

The question then becomes, "How can I stimulate the immune system to greater efficiency?" Instead of intervening with a drug treatment that ultimately *competes* with the body's natural immunity, the goal is to *complement* the natural healing mechanism. Some of the natural remedies that may assist in that goal are vitamin C (preferably the buffered, ascorbate form that the body requires), L-Lysine amino acid, and various herbs for immunity such as Echinacea and Olive Leaf. Since we're talking about infections in the lymphatic system (the body's drainage system), there are various homeopathic remedies particularly useful in stimulating the lymphatic drainage, so as to relieve congestion.

FATIGUE

Undoubtedly, fatigue is the single most common health complaint. Typically half or more of the clients entering my office list fatigue among their health concerns. No matter what the underlying causes of your health problems are, fatigue will usually be among the very first symptoms.

Unfortunately, conventional medicine isn't much help here. Normally they will run the standard Complete Blood Count (CBC) and chem-screen blood tests and tell you everything is normal, presuming no anemia showed up. The stated or unstated implication then often becomes that "It's all in your head." The truth is that hardly any of the most common causes of fatigue will show up in a conventional medical physical or blood tests.

Possible causes of fatigue that are seldom if ever addressed by conventional medicine include:

1. Food & Environmental Sensitivities – The term "sensitivity" refers to a non-specific intolerance to either a food or environmental substance. Rather than an "allergy," which refers to a specific immune system reaction, "sensitivity" describes any adverse reaction noted from exposure. The most common food sensitivity symptom is fatigue. Though, as noted in a previous chapter, a relatively small percentage of people have true medical allergies, virtually everyone has food and environmental sensitivities – it's just a question of how many one has and to what degree.

Some of the most common food sensitivities relate to grains and dairy products, though one can potentially have a sensitivity to any food. Environmental sensitivities to pollens, dust, mold, animal dander, etc. tend to be the result of *first* having food sensitivities. Ultimately food sensitivities stem from digestive issues. Foods that are not fully digested and properly assimilated tend to create sensitivities that will produce fatigue, digestive complaints, mood changes, and many other possible reactions.

Have you ever been tested for food or environmental sensitivity by your medical doctor? If you're like most, the answer would be "no." If you are among the small percentage that has had some kind of allergy testing done, it probably found next to nothing, or maybe the seemingly ever-present sensitivity to "dust mites." You, of course, weren't tested for "sensitivity," but for medical "allergy," which you're unlikely to have anyway. In most instances only a natural healing professional will test you for food and environmental **sensitivity.**

2. Nutrient Deficiencies – The various nutrients in your food are the "fuel" your body runs on. Therefore if you eat nutrient deficient food, your body will typically lack what it needs to function optimally. That will commonly manifest as fatigue, though many other health complaints might also result. Though any nutrient deficiency may contribute to fatigue, the B-vitamins are perhaps most often associated with this problem. Likewise, deficiencies of minerals such as magnesium and chromium are strongly linked to blood sugar levels, and thus commonly have a fatigue connection.

Conventional medicine will probably never test you for a nutrient deficiency, other than perhaps vitamin D, and that is only a recent development due to the enormous amount of research showing chronic vitamin D deficiency. Iron or vitamin B-12 deficiency might be inferred from a Complete Blood Count (CBC) as done by your conventional doctor, but these numbers seldom draw any action unless they are quite extreme. I would also add that the calcium test on a chem-screen blood test is actually not a test for calcium deficiency, but rather a test of parathyroid gland function. Bottom-line, you're very unlikely to ever be tested for nutrient deficiencies as a cause of fatigue by your medical doctor.

3. Toxins – With the term "toxins" I am referring to poisons and really to anything that is foreign to the body. A number of general categories of toxins exist including:

Industrial chemicals

Pesticides

Food additives

Dead bacteria or viruses

Medical drugs

Hydrocarbon-based chemicals

Heavy metals

Within these general categories tens of thousands of individual toxins exist. Understand that your body, increasingly exposed to more toxins, is created to naturally detoxify within certain limits – otherwise, none of us would be alive! But all too often the level of toxicity in a given person exceeds the body's capacity to detoxify. Initially that will produce fatigue, while later on it is likely to cause more serious health problems. As was the case with sensitivities and nutrient deficiencies, this is not something you would commonly be tested for by your medical doctor.

4. Adrenal weakness --

The adrenal glands sit on top of the kidneys and are responsible for producing hormones such as cortisol, aldosterone, DHEA, and adrenalin. Though most often associated with "fight or flight" reactions, think of the adrenals as simply releasing hormones in response to stress – *physical* stress such as infections, injuries, inflammation, toxin exposure, and the like, as well as *emotional* stress. In our present day most people live in a more or less constant state of adrenal stress. This constant "calling on" the adrenal glands to secrete stress hormones tends to result in an eventual depletion and inability to adequately respond. When the adrenals are thus exhausted, fatigue is the primary symptom. Conventional medicine rarely tests for adrenal function.

5. Thyroid weakness – Thyroid weakness likewise commonly produces fatigue, among other symptoms. Low thyroid function is often an unsuspected cause of illness, in part because of the inadequacy of standard conventional medical tests. *If* thyroid function is tested at all by your MD, it is most often done by measuring blood serum levels of T3 (Triiodothyronine), T4 (Thyroxin), and occasionally TSH (Thyroid stimulating hormone).

The problem is that all these tests measure *circulating* hormones, rather than the *cellular* levels where these hormones are actually operative. The result: A lot of false negatives, causing your doctor to say your thyroid is fine. Natural healing professionals often prefer the Basal Temperature Test, popularized by Broda Barnes, MD, as a more reliable indicator of low thyroid function. It consists of taking the axillary (under the arm) temperature with a mercury thermometer for 10 minutes the first thing when you wake up in the morning, without getting up or moving significantly. If it's below 97.8 degrees, it is suggestive of low thyroid function.

NATURAL APPROACHES TO FATIGUE

So how can you *naturally* approach the above possible causes of fatigue? Let's begin with food and environmental sensitivities. Three simple, natural things can help remedy these problems, the first being a **digestive aid**. Food and environmental sensitivities stem from insufficient digestion, as discussed previously. Getting on a compatible digestive enzyme supplement is foundational, given most people have insufficient secretions of digestive enzymes. In some cases it may also be appropriate to use a **probiotic** supplement to re-implant beneficial bacteria into the intestinal tract for more optimal function. Yet another possible approach would be a **digestive repair** supplement designed to restore the integrity of the intestinal mucosa for better function.

For the nutrient deficiency causes of fatigue, a compatible nutritional supplement is the answer. The key word here is *compatible*, since most of the nutritional supplements people take are *not* compatible with their bodies. This can be an issue of quality, given a lot of vitamin and mineral supplements people buy, particularly from supermarkets and drug stores are frankly junk. They have artificial colors, preservatives, and cheap but poorly assimilated nutrient sources such as calcium carbonate and magnesium oxide. However, compatibility is still an issue even with high quality products. Your body may "like" or "not like" a given high ingredient quality product because of particular ratios of nutrients, particular sources, something in the manufacturing method, excipients contained such as binders and fillers, or some other cause. An individualized compatibility testing method is therefore essential.

What about natural approaches for toxins? Here natural healing relies primarily on herbal and homeopathic remedies. Various herbs combat different types of infection, whether candida/fungal, bacterial, viral, or parasitic. While conventional medicine drug approaches to these problems always have side effects, the natural remedies really have none that are significant. Many different herbal remedies exist, so again it is essential to have some type of testing method for determining which are appropriate. To amplify this a little, in the testing done at my Pacific Health Center clinics we may find one or two compatible remedies out of twenty or thirty possibilities. In other words *without a specific remedy testing method*, the odds are very slim of coming up with something that will really help.

Homeopathic remedies for toxins comprise a fascinating healing possibility. Without going into an extensive explanation of homeopathic medicine, think of it as involving micro-dilutions of substances. The essential principle of homeopathy is the "like cures like," that is, a homeopathic dilution of a substance that in its normal amount *produces* ill-health symptoms, in its homeopathic dilution does the opposite – it *helps* heal the symptoms. For example, a homeopathic dilution of arsenic will stimulate the body to detoxify itself of arsenic, excreting it through the urine. A homeopathic dilution of *Candia albicans* yeast will stimulate the immune system to attack and eliminate this toxin.

Natural healing addresses low adrenal function usually with either glandular or herbal supplements. Beef adrenal gland supplements are often helpful in nourishing the human adrenal glands and thus improving their function. A number of herbs, such as Ginseng, Schisandra, Gotu kola, Ginkgo Biloba, and Licorice root, also have stimulating effects on the adrenals that in turn can translate into improved energy levels. I would add that there is a "point of no return" on damaged adrenal function. If the adrenals have altogether ceased to produce hormones (a condition called Addison 's disease), prescription drug hormone replacement will be necessary, though natural remedies can still be of some benefit.

Low thyroid function is addressed in a similar way to low adrenal function. Beef thyroid glandular supplements can stimulate the thyroid through their nutritional support, as can supplements of iodine and L-Tyrosine amino acid. Homeopathic remedies may also be helpful. In some cases natural remedies will suffice for low thyroid function, but in other cases at least some reliance on prescription drugs will be necessary.

DEPRESSION

Conventional medicine seemingly "owns" the problem of depression. Some of the largest selling prescription drugs supposedly "treat" this problem with **1 in 10 Americans taking an anti-depressant drug** – Prozac, Celexa, Effexor, Paxil, Zoloft, or others. Now think about this for a moment: Does 10% of the population really *need* to be on some drug to treat depression or is this just a great job of marketing a product? I would also note that none of these commonly used drugs has been evaluated for long-term safety; in fact, most of the studies done on them are for short-term usage rather than the very long-term usage they actually have.

The conventional medicine approach depression is just same old treating without solving the problem. You are not depressed because your body has a "deficiency" of Prozac, Paxil, or Effexor. Those drugs simply manipulate the symptoms so you feel better without actually solving any underlying cause.

As discussed earlier conventional medicine typically blames depression on a "chemical imbalance" in the brain. While that's okay so far, the error of conventional medicine is then taking the role of an interventionist, saying in effect, "There's a chemical imbalance, so let's manipulate the brain chemicals with drugs." How about asking the obvious question – **What's causing the chemical imbalance?**

The natural healing approach to depression *is* asking what is causing the chemical imbalance. Guess what? The same underlying causes show up – food & environmental sensitivities, nutrient deficiencies, toxins, and we could also add hormonal imbalances (though these are typically caused by nutrient deficiencies). Vitamin, mineral, herbal, homeopathic, or amino acid supplementation is a possible approach for addressing these root causes.

Though I've just listed three specific health problems that respond to natural healing, many others could be cited – diabetes, arthritis, fibromyalgia, digestive complaints, skin issues, headaches, cholesterol, high blood pressure, etc. We would generally find the same kinds of root causes. Natural healing usually works well, but it can also be complementary to conventional medicine in many situations.

NATURAL COMPLEMENTS CONVENTIONAL

Now let's get practical: How should natural healing be integrated together with conventional medicine? What if you're already doing conventional medicine for your health problem? Can natural healing be added in order to do a complementary approach? Usually it can be added and will be helpful.

Let's take an example: Suppose you've had your gall bladder removed. It's obviously too late to do a natural approach to heal your gall bladder, but a natural approach can help your now impaired digestion of fats and oils. This natural approach would involve a diet that minimizes fats and oils while adding in digestive enzyme supplementation. Conventional medicine alone might suggest the former, but hardly ever would suggest the latter. The complementary approach allows you to "complete what is lacking" in the conventional medicine approach alone.

I see the general rule as this:

> *Conventional medicine is usually required for problems not prevented*

Conventional medicine deals with the immediate, acute issue, while natural healing will focus more on long-term healing. This is not to say that natural healing doesn't offer alternatives for some acute situations. It indeed does offer alternatives for acute indigestion, headaches, muscle or joint pain, non-anaphylactic allergic reactions, and others, though usually a natural healing professional needs to direct such intervention. As a general rule of thumb I would propose the following:

> *Unless it is an emergency or serious acute situation, try natural healing first*

You can always fall back on conventional treatment if the natural approach is to no avail.

NATURAL HEALING CONTRAINDICATIONS

I've given examples of when natural and conventional medicine can work together in a complementary sense, but what about when they cannot? When will natural healing *not* be complementary to conventional medicine; in fact, when might natural healing even be dangerous when used with conventional medicine?

Admittedly we are talking about rather rare instances. Let me give a few examples that come to mind:

1. Organ transplantation – In this rare occurrence, immune-suppression is paramount in order to lower the risk of tissue rejection. Since natural healing methods typically *stimulate* the immune system, they could be very problematic in this instance.

2. Dialysis – This is again a relatively rare situation in terms of the number of people affected. Certain nutritional supplements would interfere with dialysis and therefore be contraindicated. These include the fat soluble vitamins – A, D, E, and K, as well as high doses of vitamin C.

3. Prescription medication conflicts with natural remedies – Some common drugs conflict with common natural remedies. Actually, perhaps *conflict* is not the right word, but rather we could say the natural remedies do the same thing as the drugs and thus can over-medicate. For example, conventional doctors with patients on the blood thinner, Coumadin, will tell their patients not to take vitamin E. Why? Well, it's simply because vitamin E also has a blood thinning effect. I would suggest, however, that given Coumadin costs four times as much as vitamin E, it might make more sense to keep the vitamin E, saying that the drug conflicts with the natural remedy rather than that the natural remedy conflicts with the drug!

Another often noted contraindication is for those taking SSRI (Selective Serotonin Re-Uptake Inhibitor) drugs for depression. They are told *not* to take L-tryptophan amino acid or St. John's Wort herb, both of which have anti-depressant effects. The logic is the same: Both the conventional drug and the natural remedy kind of do the same thing, so one may not be needed. The drug again is the expensive one with lots of side-effects, while the natural remedy is much cheaper and seldom has any side-effects.

Anti-hypertensive drugs for lowering blood pressure comprise yet another example. There are herbs, vitamins, and minerals that naturally lower blood pressure. But if you're taking a drug and the natural remedies, your blood pressure may drop too low, resulting in light-headedness or fainting. I again pose the question: If the natural remedies are that effective, maybe you don't really need the drug.

On all these types of issues it is important to ask your health practitioner, both your conventional doctor and your natural healing professional, for their perspectives. Usually the natural practitioner will at least know something about possible drug contraindications. Unfortunately most conventional medical doctors will usually not be very familiar with the natural alternatives for problems they typically prescribe drugs for. I would also add that it is very easy for anyone to check out possible contraindications of a drug or a natural remedy by simply searching it on the internet.

CONCLUSION

Conventional medicine and natural healing really can work together in many instances. However, I would hasten to add that for most common health problems, natural healing alone will usually suffice. Thus, I would emphasize the following guidelines as you consider taking the health dare:

1. Start with natural remedies unless it is an emergency or other serious acute situation.

2. Where conventional medicine is definitely needed, complement it with natural healing, if possible.

3. Do not do natural healing approaches in the rare instances where it is contraindicated.

FOOTNOTES CHAPTER SIX

1.
http://en.wikipedia.org/wiki/Wilk_v._American_Medical_Associatio
n

2. http://www.cdc.gov/getsmart/antibiotic-use/know-and-do.html

3. http://www.mayoclinic.org/healthy-living/consumer-health/in-depth/antibiotics/art-20045720

Chapter 7
Natural Healing is Life-Changing

Is natural healing really life-changing? Let me explain how natural healing changed my life and can change yours. In the first chapter I shared my experience with cancer, but there's another "angle" to the story. Yes, conventional medicine destroyed my health while supposedly "treating" my disease. Yes, a combination of natural approaches rebuilt my health and kept me cancer-free for the past 40 years. But it really wasn't as simple as just going to a different *kind* of doctor and having him *solve* my cancer problem.

My experience with natural healing for cancer indeed changed my life, but **it was life-changing because I was forced to change my life.** Under the conventional cancer approach I was a patient being treated. With the natural healing approach I was a participant pursuing healing. If you take the "health dare" of trying natural healing, it will impose some lifestyle changes that will transform your life and health.

Natural healing is distinctly different in this way. While conventional medicine lets you be passive (or often insists you be passive), that really doesn't work with natural healing. You have to become fully engaged and take charge. I had to first learn, by doing a lot of reading, a different approach to dealing with a degenerative disease. I had to take a lot of nutritional supplements. I had to eat a strict diet. I had to exercise to stimulate my circulation and resultant healing. Overall, I had to adopt a number of disciplines that no doctor could do for me. My doctor was a teacher, and I was a student. Let's look more specifically at how natural healing does change your life.

PATIENT VS. PARTICIPANT

Education provides an interesting parallel with conventional versus natural healing. Contemporary education is rather pathetic in my view. It's what one of my professors called the "storage tank approach" – just transferring the contents from one brain to another with no real critical thinking.

Much of education today is not really education, but rather *indoctrination* – essentially propaganda. Most schools, from elementary school to medical school, just teach you to memorize someone else's opinion. The *educator* becomes an outside agent **doing something to you** in your passivity. Ultimately the goal is not so much to truly *know* something, but just to get a diploma – what my college roommate referred to as a [expletive deleted] *ticket*.

Historic education was considerably different from most of what goes on today. Back then the main objective was to teach you to *think*. The teacher's job was to motivate you to internally process information, rather than just memorizing a bunch of supposed "facts." Therefore, you ultimately taught yourself. In my view all true education is ultimately *self-education*, though teachers are involved in motivating that process. Contemporary education asks, "Where did you go to school?" while historic education asks, "What do you know?" and "Who did you study under?"

So how's this relate to health care? Conventional medicine follows pretty much the same pattern as our indoctrination-propaganda educational system. It's something they *do* to you. You are the passive one whom they "treat," rather than "teach" a healthy lifestyle to.

Natural medicine not only doesn't work that way, but it *won't* work that way. It requires you to be the primary implementer of the program, not the doctor. The program is not just take this pill till the bottle is empty or have this surgery, but rather is **live this way**. Now we're talking about a 24/7 activity, so the "doctor" can't do all that for you.

Let me hasten to add that natural healing requires a certain kind of subject. Some people are thoroughly programmed by their conventional medicine experience toward passivity, coming into the doctor's office with a "Doctor, heal me" attitude. They don't really want to take responsibility for their health care. Natural healing demands a person that wants to dig in and solve their problems – a person not so much interested in being "treated" as in being "taught" how to be healthy.

UNCHANGED LIFESTYLE

Not wanting to participate in one's health care is, however, only half of the problem. An equally significant problem is the person who just doesn't want to change. Mind you, they want their health problem solved, but they want to keep their present lifestyle – kind of a "have your cake and eat it too" approach. If that's where you're at, you are an ideal candidate for conventional medicine, but you're way too lazy for natural healing.

I could share examples galore of things conventional medicine patients actually (and unbelievably do):

> After the triple bypass eating diet high in trans fats
>
> Insulin-dependent diabetic eating refined sugar
>
> Sinus/allergy sufferer on antihistamines drinking milk
>
> PMS/menopausal woman eating caffeine and dairy
>
> After throat cancer surgery smoking a cigarette through the tracheotomy hole in the neck

The message is basically, "Take this pill or have this surgery and live however you please." Of course, that may not be explicitly said, but it is nevertheless implied since seldom is any lifestyle change suggested. The end result is simply trading one health problem for another. You treat one set of symptoms, but you did nothing to resolve the underlying problem, often ending up with an even worse problem.

THE CURSE OF IATROGENESIS

Though it's bad enough that the root cause is typically not dealt with in conventional medicine, the often greater problem is that of *iatrogenic disease* – that is, "doctor-caused" disease. If the "treatment" produces another health problem, we call it iatrogenic. If you take statin drugs for cholesterol and get muscle achiness from the drug decreasing your Co-enzyme Q10 levels, that's iatrogenic. If you take acetaminophen for pain and thus damage your liver, that's iatrogenic. If your gall bladder is surgically removed producing greater indigestion, that's iatrogenic. And on the list goes.

Most conventional treatments, unfortunately, result in some kind of iatrogenesis. That's the price you pay for treating symptoms instead of resolving underlying causes.

PRINCIPLE OF REPENTANCE

Though you may think of "repentance" as a religious or theological term, it actually plays right into to our topic. To "repent" simply means to change directions. You were going south and you turn around and go north instead. A lot of people need to make this kind of "180" with their health. But this is not a new problem. There's an interesting story in the Bible concerning a man with a health problem that required a lifestyle change. After healing a paralytic man at the Pool of Bethesda, Jesus said:

> *See, you are well! Sin no more; that nothing worse may happen to you.* (John 5:14b)

Here's my fantasy: Imagine more conventional medicine doctors doing that with their patients and saying things like:

> *If you don't want another bypass, quit eating sugar and trans fats.*

> *If you don't want another kidney stone operation, start drinking distilled water and balance out your mineral metabolism.*

If you don't want cancer again, quit eating food full of hormones and chemicals.

True healing assumes a cause. Your problem didn't just "happen." As King Solomon wrote:

The curse causeless shall not come. (Proverbs 26:2b, KJV)

So what am I saying? If you want to *stay* healed, your behavior must change – there's no free lunch. To change your health, you must change your life, including what you eat and drink, your exercise, your sleep, and your handling of stress, to name a few. Changing your lifestyle improves your overall health by preventing the next problem.

STEP BY STEP CHANGES

For most people the best lifestyle changes are made gradually. Of course, it doesn't always work out that way for some of us. In my cancer experience it was strictly "cold turkey." One day I was eating a fairly typical American diet, while the next day we were trying to figure out how to eat raw foods, no meat, and a bunch of other changes. That was hard for a while, but I really was desperate, plus I really believed the direction my nutritionally-oriented MD gave me was sound. Focus on these steps:

1. Diet – The biggest challenge is usually dietary change. Since my difficult time converting to a healthier diet to deal with cancer decades ago, I have learned how to make that transition a lot easier. I wrote *The Junk Food Withdrawal Manual*[1] to show others how. The concept is summed up in two principles:

1. Substitution rather than deprivation using nine easy health food substitutions

2. Gradual transition with a 12-week "withdrawal" program

2. Supplements & Remedies – This is a big deal or a small deal depending on what you're accustomed to. To some people, taking one multi-vitamin pill a day is a huge imposition. To someone else that's been using supplements a long time, taking six or eight different products daily is routine.

Most of the negative reaction people have to "taking vitamins" comes from equating these natural remedies with drugs. Yes, both prescription drugs and vitamins come in pills or capsules, but that's where the similarities end. Vitamins, mineral, enzymes, amino acids, etc. *actually belong in your body*. Chemical drugs, on the other hand, are quite foreign to your body, and thus your body treats them as toxins, trying to eliminate them through the liver, kidneys, and other elimination pathways.

What should freak you out is the thought of taking six or eight different prescription *drugs* daily – things that really don't belong in your body – not taking in supplemental nutrients that *should be* in your body (and would be in your body if you ate an optimal diet). Unless you want to take those highly toxic, symptom-treating drugs and suffer their side-effects, you need to take some nutritional supplements and other natural remedies. You don't have to take a hundred pills a day, but you aren't going to resolve any significant health problems taking a cheap, inorganic, pharmaceutical company multi-vitamin (that your body probably can't even digest) either. If you have hang-ups in this area, I suggest you get over them, or you're really not a candidate for natural healing.

3. Exercise – Our bodies were created to be active. Few things damage health as much as simply sitting around doing nothing. Recent studies indicate that simply sitting for a long period of time, without getting up every few minutes and moving around, greatly damages health. We all know what happens to a tool, a piece of machinery or a car that isn't used. Whether it's rust, damage from lack of lubrication, or other causes, that item just isn't as good as one used regularly. Do you think your body is any different?

Having said that, I'm not keen on most "exercise" programs, in that I believe physical work is the best exercise. I encourage my clients to stop *avoiding* work. My motto is, "Walk, don't ride." Walk wherever it is practical and possible within your physical abilities. Walk up a stairs instead of taking an elevator (provided we're not talking about a skyscraper). Do your own yard work, but again don't exceed your particular physical limitations. Take up gardening, if you're not already doing that. Go hiking in the summer and cross-country skiing in the winter. Be creative as you consider possibilities for bringing meaningful, practical physical work into your life. Do enough of that and you won't need formal "exercise."

4. Individualized Health Program – The ultimate step in changing to a healthier lifestyle is some kind of individualized health program. It is a fundamental truth that we are all different. When it comes to our health problems, we have different causes and therefore different solutions. The old saying, "One man's meat is another man's poison," is really quite true.

Regrettably, most people simply guess at what's going to help their health, with little to no factual data to guide them. Sometimes this is simply a matter of pride, where one wants the ego satisfaction of "figuring out" their health situation all by themselves. The "Do-It-Yourselfer" reads about all kinds of health problems and remedies and then goes to the discount vitamin store, online, or in response to a slick mail order piece to get what they think will be their "cure." Usually they only waste their time and money, just as I did the first time, as a teenager, walking into this weird place called a "health food store" without a clue as to what I needed.

Instead of the "pride" approach above, may I suggest the "humility" approach? Admit that you don't know what you're doing and go to a professional that does. I could try to fix my car, as I used to when I was younger, but it's so much more effective when I take it to a professional that actually knows what's going on. Let's acknowledge the "division of labor." We don't all do everything. We're not all knowledgeable in everything. We're not all skilled in fixing everything. So, make a living at what you're good at and trained for, but get help from others for the areas outside your expertise, particularly when it comes to your health.

I wish I could say that when you get "professional help" in the health arena, it will be based on individual testing of your body. However, that is often *not* the case. While the average person gets their ideas about health and remedies mostly from media inputs, often doctors aren't much better. Even the natural healing doctors most often use what I call a "textbook" approach to designing a healing program. For example, if you're fatigued, the textbook says you probably need B-vitamins, so they try that. If you're depressed, the textbook says that tryptophan is a good remedy, so they try that, and on it goes. The problem is that this is simply educated guessing and is not based on any actual assessment of what your body needs.

My own 30+ year practice has always focused on individualized testing, since that was the only thing that made sense to me. I never wanted to treat symptoms, but rather to strive to understand the likely underlying causes of a health problem. Specifically, I built my practice around discovering and correcting three "common denominators" of most health problems:

Food & Environmental Sensitivity

Nutrient Deficiencies

Toxins

No matter what your *specific* problem is, I've found that most health issues come down to these three. Instead of having a different program or protocol for every diagnostic category under the sun, I simply identify and correct these three, thus freeing up the body to heal itself as God intended.

We're really good at making things complicated, aren't we? I like to keep things simple, so here's an even simpler (and life-changing) way of looking at your health. Simply ask yourself these two questions about your body:

What's missing (that should be there)?

What's present (that should *not* be there)?

"What's missing" speaks to the realm of nutrient deficiencies, while "what's present" concerns sensitivities and toxins. Then all you really need to ask is which remedies are the right ones to correct what's missing and what's present. What remedies are actually *compatible* and *effective* for your body? An individual testing method will answer those questions. Whether you use my individual testing method or some other method, I would simply emphasize that you need *some* kind of individual testing (more information on my testing is found in the Appendix).

CONCLUSION

Natural healing both changes your life *and* requires you to make lifestyle changes to experience its full benefits. In this regard, natural healing is very different from most conventional medicine that all too often separates behavior from health problems. It's not an overstatement to say that our health problems flow from our lifestyle. Therefore, to change your health, change your life. The "health dare" of natural healing will help you do just that.

Yet a deeper question remains: Is there an ultimate design for good health? Does God have a way that we can learn, apply, and derive the benefits from? That's our final topic in our health dare.

CHAPTER SEVEN FOOTNOTES

1. Kline, Monte, *The Junk Food Withdrawal Manual*, www.pacifichealthcenter.com.

Chapter 8

Natural Healing Reflects God's Design

Have you ever had an appliance that was not working correctly and found yourself looking for the Owner's Manual? I do that rather regularly when it comes to programming my office phones – "Now which buttons do I push to save a phone number?" If something doesn't work, we tend to want to find the instructions to figure out what's wrong. There is always a right way and usually a lot of wrong ways of doing something, whether it's operating a computer, fixing your car, transplanting tomatoes in the garden, preparing a recipe for dinner, or whatever.

Now what about your body? Can't we also assume there is a right and wrong way of "operating" it? If it's not working correctly – that is, you have a health problem – isn't it logical to assume you haven't been following the Manufacturer's instructions? The highly unlikely alternative, of course, is to assume that your body just happened, that lightning struck a puddle of muck making life happen out of nothing, followed by billions of years of gradual transformation into higher life forms. That's faith in an unprovable theory to the extreme.

Well, if you believe that, good luck. I gave up on that view of life as a geology major in college, since I didn't have enough "religious" faith to believe in such a far-fetched story. But for some, even concocting a wild theory is better than believing you did not just happen out of randomness. Design always points to designer. When I look out my window at my garage, I know it didn't happen from some random act, but rather there was a plan and thus a planner. The same is true of my house, my car, the desk I'm sitting at, the computer I'm typing at, and about anything I can see. Things don't just happen. If that's true of everything around you, wouldn't it also be true of your body?

If you assume as a "creation" that you had a "Creator," the next step is to check out the "Owner's Manual" in order to optimize your health. However, let me emphasize that I'm not *just* talking about the Bible, though it does have some amazing things to say about health. I would start at an even more basic level – simply observing how your body was created to function.

As we make this final consideration in my "health dare," the critical point is to determine which approach to health best "lines up" with our created design: Is it conventional medicine or natural health care?

GOD'S DESIGN – AUTOMATIC HEALING

Of the many things we often take for granted, automatic healing must be near the top of the list. Our bodies are under continual assault from millions of germs, and yet, most of the time we don't get sick. If you cut your finger, you probably don't worry about bleeding to death, but why not? After all, if a blood vessel is broken, why wouldn't it logically just keep bleeding? If you overdo working or playing sports causing you to be stiff and lame, do you expect that to be the condition for the rest of your life? Of course not! So what is it that we take for granted with our bodies? Automatic healing.

Our bodies were created to *automatically heal*, at least within certain limits. God gave us an immune system and various other mechanisms that take care of routine illnesses, injuries and the like. You don't have to think about it or will it to happen – it just automatically happens. Apart from that every one of us would probably be dead within days. This is just the way we were made.

COOPERATING OR COMPETING?

Because God's design is automatic healing, we would then infer that his design is likewise to **help the natural healing** process. The main question, then, is simply:

Do we cooperate or compete with the automatic healing process built in to our bodies?

If automatic healing is really the way life functions, we obviously should find ways to cooperate with it rather than interfering with it. So, how do the different healing approaches stack up with this measure?

Conventional medicine often *does* rely on automatic healing. Your doctor may bandage a laceration, but he or she is depending on the body to automatically heal. The antiseptic, the bandage, the stiches, if needed, *cooperate* with the natural healing process built in to the body. The same is true with a broken bone. The doctor presumes the bone will automatically heal, but setting the bone straight enhances that process and produces the most favorable outcome.

This is all well and good, but conventional medicine also commonly *competes* with natural healing. Before I give several examples of the damage this competition does, understand the root motivation for doctors competing with automatic healing is simply what I call "White Horse Syndrome." The doctor takes an interventionist approach in order to be the hero riding in on a white horse. The doctor practicing "heroic medicine" is trained to rescue and save you. Invariable the doctor takes on a "god role" in this scenario.

I think this "heroic" view of doctors probably reached its apex when I was a kid in the 1950's and 1960's. It was the era of wonder drugs and surgery for whatever ailed you. The doctors were the high priests of the religion of modern medicine, while the patient was the lowly peon feeling so privileged to get a few minutes of time with the "health oracle" who would serve the "sacrament" of prescription drugs. And the Mayo Clinic, at least for those of us living in the Midwest, was Jerusalem. This was before anyone knew much about iatrogenic (doctor-caused) disease and malpractice suits were rare. To really get an idea of that time period's exalted view of doctors, just watch Rock Hudson & Jane Wyman in the 1954 movie, "The Magnificent Obsession," where Dr. Merrick is practically worshipped in the final, very emotional climax of the film.

Recalling the resulting medical arrogance of those times, I occasionally like to repeat the Camel cigarette commercial of that time with its famous line:

More doctors smoke Camels than any other cigarette

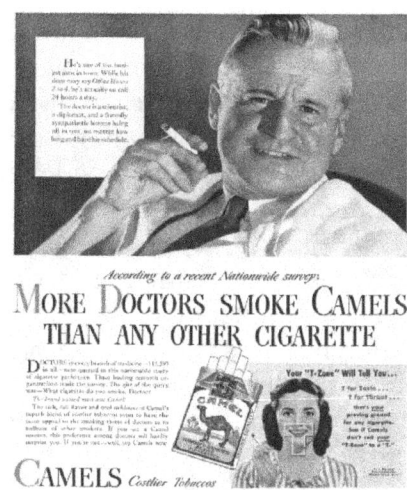

According to a recent Nationwide survey:

MORE DOCTORS SMOKE CAMELS
THAN ANY OTHER CIGARETTE

CAMELS *Costlier Tobaccos*

A well-known doctor of the time was once quoted saying:

A pack of Camels a day keeps lung cancer away

Anyway, that reminder is my suggested "cure" when conventional medicine gets a little too high and mighty when riding in to rescue you from your health problems!

ANTIBIOTIC COMPETITION

The arrogance of the "heroic medicine" approach causes a lot of problems – a lot of **health** problems. Let's take antibiotic usage, for example. For over 50 years most doctors have given out antibiotic drugs like candy, failing to recognize one can get too much of a good thing. We all acknowledge that antibiotics have saved millions of lives from diseases that were previously untreatable. Generally we could say the principle behind antibiotic therapy is consistent with God's design. But when doctors started giving antibiotics for every little infection they encountered, a whole host of *new* health problems were created.

Antibiotics are rather indiscriminate in their working, as referred to in Chapter Six – they kill "bad" bacteria, but also "good" bacteria. You have to understand that "bacteria" are not categorically bad, but rather are essential to health. Beneficial intestinal bacteria such as *Lactobacillus acidophilus* and others provide important immunity to infections such as *Candida albicans* yeast overgrowth. Before antibiotics, one hardly, if ever, heard of a systemic yeast infection, but today it is one of the most common issues confronted by natural healing practitioners (with much of conventional medicine still in denial). The condition is almost entirely *iatrogenic* – doctor-caused. When you kill off both the good and bad bacteria taking an antibiotic, you destroy a significant part of your immune system that would normally prevent such yeast overgrowth.

Do you ever wonder why today we have, particularly in children, deaths from exposure to *E. coli*, such as a number of years ago with the well-publicized case concerning a Jack in the Box fast-food restaurant? Is our food supply really more contaminated with harmful bacteria than it was 50 or 100 years ago? I doubt it. In fact, I suspect our food supply is considerably cleaner than in times past. So what has changed? Could it be that the average kid has been so bombarded with antibiotic drugs for every little infection that they lack the normal immunity to deal with an occasional *E. coli* bacteria? I don't definitely know this to be the cause, but it sure makes a lot of sense to me.

This wouldn't be quite so bad if antibiotics were properly used for the only thing they actually help – **bacterial infections**. The fact of the matter is that a significant percentage of medical doctors give antibiotics for **viral infections**, even though everyone knows antibiotics only kill bacteria and have no effect on viruses. Major health organizations, recognizing the damage this causes, for years have campaigned against this over-usage of antibiotics. On the Centers for Disease Control (CDC) webpage entitled, "Antibiotic Resistance Questions & Answers," the following is stated:

> *Antibiotic use promotes development of antibiotic-resistant bacteria. Every time a person takes antibiotics, sensitive bacteria are killed, but resistant germs may be left to grow and multiply. Repeated and improper uses of antibiotics are primary causes of the increase in drug-resistant bacteria.*[1]

In my view the proper usage of antibiotics is to reserve them for very serious or life-threatening infections. If you thus rarely use antibiotics, they're a lot more likely to work in such a situation.

THE CURSE OF CHEMOTHERAPY

Conventional medicine has three basic cancer "treatments" (if you want to call them that): surgery, radiation, and chemotherapy, or as it is known in natural healing circles – cut, burn, and poison. All three of these supposed cancer "treatments" ironically, can actually *cause* cancer! Somehow that seems rather inconsistent with God's design for health. Beyond that rather major objection, chemotherapy kills *both* cancer cells and healthy cells, resulting in horrendous side-effects. This fact prompted Allen Levin, MD of UC San Francisco to state in his book *The Healing of Cancer*:

> *Most cancer patients in this country die of chemotherapy. Chemotherapy does not eliminate breast, colon, or lung cancers. This fact has been documented for over a decade, yet doctors still use chemotherapy for these tumors.* [2]

The ineffectiveness of chemotherapy is further echoed by Thomas Dao, MD in the *New England Journal of* Medicine:

> *Despite widespread use of chemotherapies, breast cancer mortality has not changed in the last 70 years* [3]

Dr. Charles Moertal of the Mayo Clinic states:

> *Our most effective regimens are fraught with risks and side-effects and practical problems; and after this price is paid by all the patients we have treated, only a small fraction are rewarded with a transient period of usually incomplete tumor regressions .* [4]

It's the same story: competing with the body's natural healing mechanisms rather than cooperating with them.

MAMMOGRAM DANGERS

Prescribing mammograms for routine cancer screening is an article of faith in conventional medicine. The theory has always been that having a mammogram allows your doctor to catch your cancer early enough to successfully treat it. A study at Aarhus University in Denmark debunks this. Mammograms allow *seeing* a lot of cancers that are unlikely to develop into serious problems, but nevertheless trigger the whole "cut, burn, poison" (surgery, radiation, chemotherapy) response from conventional medicine. Mammograms are a great marketing tool for "selling" conventional cancer treatment, but they are of very questionable healing value. The Danish study found the same number of aggressive, late-stage breast cancer cases **with or without mammograms!** Basically, mammograms *cause more treatment* but *don't decrease overall mortality* from the disease. One of the most recent studies, as reported in the *New York Times*, noted:

> *One of the largest and most meticulous studies of mammography ever done, involving 90,000 women and lasting a quarter-century, has added powerful new doubts about the value of the screening test for women of any age. It found that the death rates from breast cancer and from all causes were the same in women who got mammograms and those who did not. And the screening had harms: one in five cancers found with mammography and treated was not a threat to the woman's health and did not need treatment such as chemotherapy, surgery or radiation.*[5]

In 2014 the Swiss Medical Board, after extensive study, recommended that no new systematic mammography screening programs to introduced and existing ones phased out. They noted that breast cancer death is only prevented in one woman in 1000, while many more are harmed.[6]

So how does this problem occur? It's pretty simple: The mammogram will show lots of false positives – "abnormalities" that are insignificant and would either go away by themselves or would never lead to a serious cancer condition. Likewise, the radiation of the mammogram, in and of itself, is carcinogenic, leading Russell Blaylock, MD to note that annual mammograms increase a woman's odds of getting breast cancer 2% each year.[7]

As with all these examples, the point is simple: When you compete with the body's God-designed natural healing mechanisms, you cause more health problems.

THE UNASKED QUESTION

It seems that conventional medicine seldom asks this key question:

What is the body doing in this illness, and how can I help it?

How do you cooperate with the body as it is dealing with an infection? How do you cooperate with the body dealing with cancer? When is intervention appropriate, and when does it make the problem worse?

NATURAL VS. CONVENTIONAL

The official name for conventional medicine is *allopathy*, literally meaning "against disease." Thus by definition, conventional medicine focuses on attacking disease rather than building health. By contrast, natural healing's main focus is just the opposite – building health rather than attacking disease.

Natural healing builds health specifically by detoxifying the body and providing essential nutrients. When your body is sick, it is toxic. Thus, a detoxification program cooperates with healing, encouraging the body to do what it is already doing through its built-in, automatic healing mechanisms. All health ultimately revolves around cellular nourishment – if the cells are properly nourished you'll be healthy; if they're not, you won't. Natural healing asks what nutrients are outright missing from the body, or what *extra* nutrients, beyond normal requirements, will further healing.

This contrast is further complicated by the *effects* of each healing approach. It is one thing to say that conventional medicine approaches healing this way, and natural healing approaches it another way, but what is the result of each approach? What are the unintended consequences?

Simply stated, most conventional healing approaches have undesirable side-effects, as referred to earlier in our discussion of antibiotics, chemotherapy, and mammography. In other words you "treat" one problem, but end up with additional new health problems requiring further treatment, as referred to in "The American Death Ceremony" in Chapter Five.

By contrast, natural healing methods have no significant side-effects beyond a possible minor discomfort that some experience during detoxification. By focusing on root causes rather than attacking the outward symptoms, positive results are often slower in coming, yet deliver a much better long-term outcome.

Though it may seem somewhat presumptuous to present "God's Design" in healing, I believe simply looking at the way we're created affirms such truths. Using the foundation of the automatic healing we all experience every day, it is no great stretch to observe that conventional, symptom-attacking medicine typically "competes" with this built-in healing process, while natural healing seeks to cooperate with it by resolving underlying root causes. I can think of no better reason to take the "health dare" of trying natural healing.

CHAPTER 8 FOOTNOTES

1. http://www.cdc.gov/getsmart/antibiotic-use/antibiotic-resistance-faqs.html#bacteria-viruses

2. http://www.cancertutor.com/deathbydoctoring4/

3. *New England Journal of Medicine*, March 1975, 292, p. 707.

4. http://www.cancertutor.com/deathbydoctoring4/

5. *New York Times*, February 11, 2014.

6. Swiss Medical Board, December 15, 2013, "Systematic Mammography Screening."

7. draxe.com/mammograms-cause-cancer/

Closing Thoughts

I began this book "daring" you to try natural healing. Unlike most dares, however, this dare was based on a solid foundation of facts. Though it would seem logical that most people would try natural healing out of pure common sense, other interfering factors are in play.

For our whole lives we have been bombarded with pro-conventional medicine propaganda through the media, schools, church, friends, parents and the like. Conventional medicine is definitely the "establishment" view of health, and the prime focus of any establishment is to maintain its preeminent position. It's not easy to break away from this intense pressure to conform, and thus, I had to "dare" you to try another path to health.

But a paradigm shift is occurring today relative to health care, simply because more and more people are recognizing that conventional medicine doesn't work very well for at least most chronic health problems. Like the fairy tale of the Emperor whose subjects were propagandized into praising the naked Emperor's clothes, many of us are becoming the little boy who honestly proclaims, "The Emperor has no clothes!"

Conventional medicine has a lot of things: respect, huge institutions, favored status with the government and insurance companies, and money, but it lacks the most important thing – results. It creates perhaps as many health problems as it solves through iatrogenesis and yet still maintains its respected position.

What will change this? What will finally complete the paradigm shift back to historic, natural healing? You will. You and millions more who educate themselves about healing. You who dare to try natural healing and experience its life-changing value.

About the Author

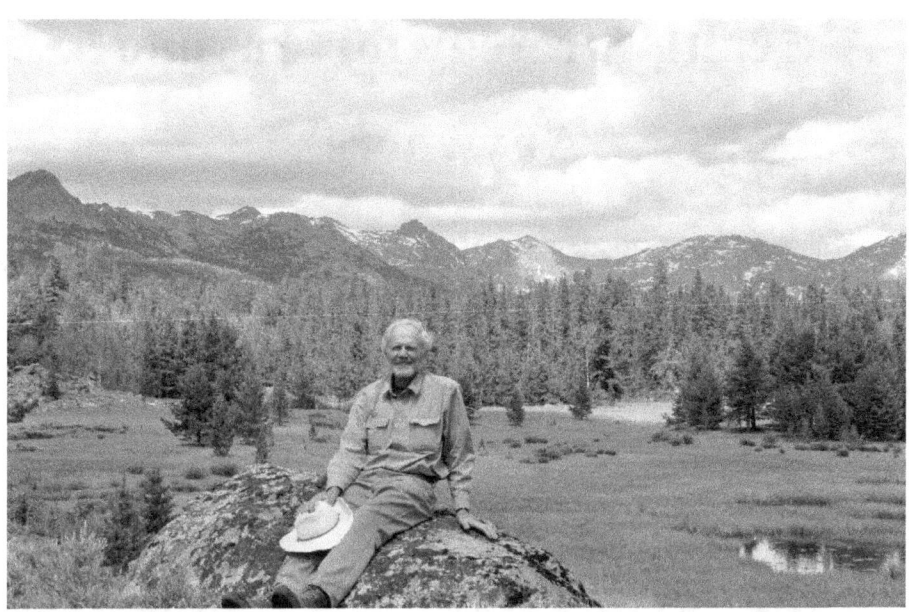

After growing up in the Midwest, Monte Kline came to the Pacific Northwest in pursuit of a college education in geology and to enjoy the region's scenic beauty. However, coming to know Christ his sophomore year changed his plans, redirecting him after graduation into several years of college campus Christian ministry. During that time he developed a serious cancer condition that was ultimately resolved with a natural medicine approach. This experience launched him into a career of speaking, writing books and presenting health and nutrition from a biblical perspective, including *Eat, Drink & Be Ready, The Junk Food Withdrawal Manual, Vitamin Manual for the Confused, The Sick & Tired Manual, Body, Mind & Health* and *Face to Face*. After completing a graduate degree in Nutrition & Wholistic Health Sciences, Monte went into practice as a Clinical Nutritionist in 1984. He currently directs two Pacific Health Center practices in the Northwest.

Monte, along with his wife Nancy live near Sisters, Oregon.

Monte may be contacted regarding speaking engagements or his clinical practice at **drkline@pacifichealthcenter.com** or Pacific Health Center, PO Box 1066, Sisters, OR 97759.

Appendix A – Physical Health
A Health Strategy for Anyone . . . Anywhere

As discussed in this book, health involves several "common denominator" factors including:

Food & environmental sensitivities

Nutrient deficiencies

Toxins

Organ stress

Compatible natural remedies

Ultimately, we must have answers to two fundamental questions:

1. What's *missing* in my body (that should be there)?

2. What's *present* in my body (that should not be there)?

Thus, our health approach is then to put the good into the body and remove the bad. But how does one answer those questions? How do you find out "what's missing" and "what's present," so as to free up your body's natural healing processes?

Enter **Remote Health Screening** or what we like to call **E-Health.** Pacific Health Center tests clients, not only at our local Oregon offices, but literally all over the world with our custom designed Zyto technology program featuring:

1. Remote testing through a "Hand Cradle" plugged into your PC computer:

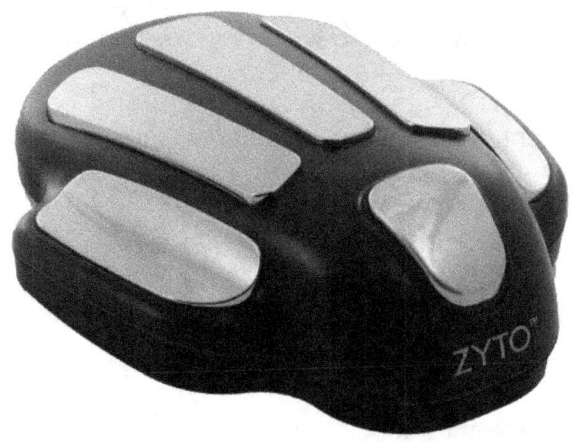

2. Non-invasively measures changes in galvanic skin resistance in response to thousands of "virtual stressors and balancers" – essentially computer signatures that simulate exposure to an item.

3. Assessing "common denominators" of all health problems – food & environmental sensitivities, nutrient deficiencies, toxins, stressed organs, and compatible natural remedies.

4. Remote connection to Pacific Health Center through the internet, while talking by phone or Skype and observing testing computer screen through screen sharing – just as in in the office as shown below:

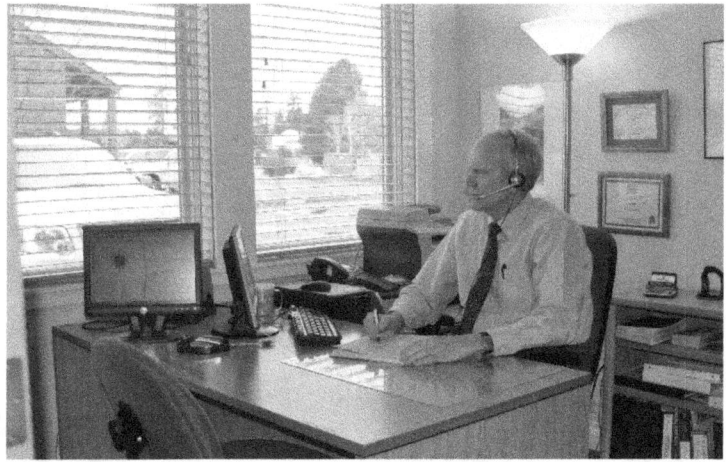

Pacific Health Center's approach, along with a demonstration of the remote, "E-Health" screening, may be viewed in the Free **SICK & TIRED WEBINAR** at the following link:

http://www.pacifichealthcenter.com/client-webinar-signup-recorded.html

You may also schedule a Free Health Screening Telephone Consultation with Monte Kline to discuss your health issues at the following link:

http://www.pacifichealthcenter.com/health-screening.html

We look forward to helping you to better health . . . naturally.

-- *Monte Kline, Clinical Nutritionist*

Discover Health in Body, Mind and Spirit

The Bible recognizes that we are body, mind and spirit, but how does that relate to our everyday health? How do we discover our physical, emotional and spiritual ingredients of health? Simply by going back to God's design. Our Creator is in the business of producing wholeness in body, mind and spirit. We are "healthy" when we are "whole." Our health problems therefore stem from the "holes" in our "wholeness." What physical ingredients of health are you missing? What emotional ingredients? What spiritual ingredients? BODY, MIND & HEALTH probes these questions providing practical answers through nutrition, detoxification, exercise, emotional stress release, and spiritual renewal.

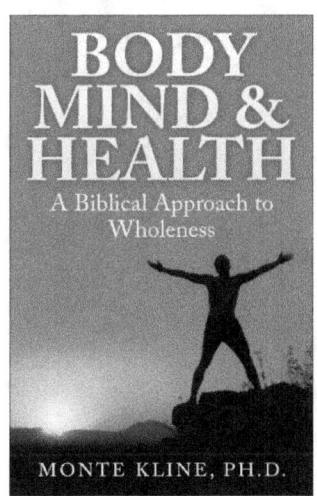

Chapters:

Your Health Checklist
God-Made Food
Water that Refreshes
Cleansing that Purifies
By the Sweat of Your Brow

Let the Sun Shine
Sleep that Satisfies
Healthy Attitudes
Capturing the Present Moment
Resolving Emotional Stress
Spiritual Roadblocks to Health
Defeating Spiritual Strongholds
Total Health at the Cross
Living in God's Sovereignty

Excellent book. I learned a lot from reading it. The author has really done his research. One of the key things I learned from this book is that healing comes from many sources such as emotional, spiritual, and mental, not just the physical aspect, which tends to be the one aspect that most people tend to focus on. Very enlightening. I highly recommend it -- Shawn Clark

Order at this link: **http://www.amazon.com/dp/B00M9TFQKE**

Appendix C – Emotional & Spiritual Health

Encounter God through Personal Retreats

Dealing with the "missing ingredients" of *physical health* is one thing, but what about your emotional and spiritual health? How do you bring healing to those areas? My suggestion: Have an **encounter with God** – what I call a **Personal Retreat**.

Has God spoken to you lately? Imagine a whole new way of meeting with God that would transform your Christian life. What if you could create special times alone with God for illumination, direction on decisions, and just the sheer enjoyment of being in His presence . . . like nothing you ever experienced before? What if you could come "face to face" with God? My book, *Face to Face: Meeting God in the Quiet Places* provides the blueprint. Following the pattern of Abraham, Elijah, Paul, and Jesus, *Face to Face* shows the way to create those life-changing encounters. You will discover:

A way to meet with God and hear his voice

Keys to escaping the "noise" and busyness of life

An alternative to "Christmas list" praying

How to "capture" your spiritual transformation

How to encounter God through Personal Retreats

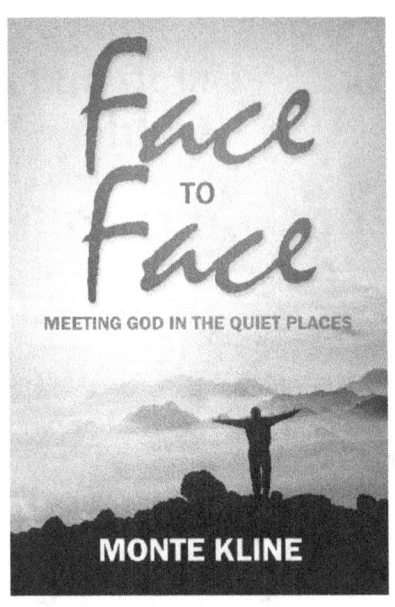

What others say . . .

> **Face to Face** *lays out a game plan for a deeper and more meaningful relationship with Christ.* – Tom Flick, Motivational Speaker and former NFL quarterback

> *Only you and Him. It stands to reason you need some quality time* **Face to Face.** – Stu Weber, Author of Tender Warrior

Order at this link: **http://www.amazon.com/dp/B00M1ZBIU8**

www.ingramcontent.com/pod-product-compliance
Lightning Source LLC
Chambersburg PA
CBHW070924290526
45795CB00001B/414